Powers of Abjection

In this book, Ricardo Laleff Ilieff presents a new ontological understanding of politics through the writings of Julia Kristeva's notion of "abjection" in dialogue with Sigmund Freud's concept of "Unheimlich" and Jacques Lacan's ontology "du réel".

Aimed at those who are interested in the politics-psychoanalytic "praxis", Laleff Ilieff argues that the abject enables one to critically read conceptual developments that are central to contemporary thought. Examining the abject in sacrifice, war, and the One as articulated by contemporary thinkers such as Walter Benjamin, Judith Butler, Carl Schmitt, René Girard, Pierre Clastres, Giorgio Agamben, and Jacques Rancière, Laleff Ilieff argues that abjection does not operate on the margins of the social but is what unveils the failure of all identity.

Powers of Abjection provides new questions and insights into the relation between psychoanalysis and politics and is an invaluable resource to students and scholars.

Ricardo Laleff Ilieff is Professor of Political Theory at the Gino Germani Research Institute (University of Buenos Aires) as well as a researcher at the National Council for Scientific and Technical Research (CONICET) of Argentina.

Psychoanalytic Political Theory
Edited by Matthew H. Bowker
University at Buffalo
and David W. McIvor
Colorado State University

Psychoanalytic Political Theory provides a publishing space for the highest quality scholarship at the intersection of psychoanalysis and normative political theory. It offers a forum for texts that deepen our understanding of the complex relationships between the world of politics and the world of the psyche.

Recently Published Books

2. **Individuality and Ideology in British Object Relations Theory**
   Gal Gerson

3. **The Psychopathology of Political Ideologies**
   Robert Samuels

4. **Psychoanalysis Under Occupation**
   Practicing Resistance in Palestine
   Stephen Sheehi and Lara Sheehi

5. **Revisiting State Personhood and World Politics**
   Identity, Personality, and the IR subject
   Bianca Naude

6. **Winnicott and Labor's Eclipse of Life**
   Work is Where We Start From
   Nathan Gerard

7. **Rethinking Property**
   Drive Theory, Fanon, and Environmental Philosophy
   Elliott Schwebach

8. **Powers of Abjection**
   Politics and Lacanian Ontology
   Ricardo Laleff Ilieff

Powers of Abjection

Politics and Lacanian Ontology

Ricardo Laleff Ilieff

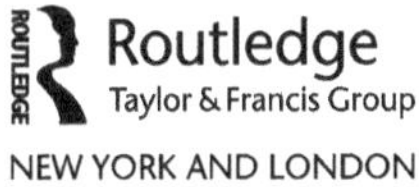

NEW YORK AND LONDON

First published in English, 2025
by Routledge
605 Third Avenue, New York, NY 10158

and by Routledge
4 Park Square, Milton Park, Abingdon, Oxon, OX14 4RN

Routledge is an imprint of the Taylor & Francis Group, an informa business

Published in Spanish by Miño y Davila Editores, 2023

ISBN: 978-1-032-59967-0 (hbk)
ISBN: 978-1-032-59968-7 (pbk)
ISBN: 978-1-003-45702-2 (ebk)

DOI: 10.4324/9781003457022

Typeset in Times New Roman
by Apex CoVantage, LLC

To Mandela Muniagurria, for her love,
her support and company;
for our conversations and readings;
for the limitless possibilities of this list.

Contents

Acknowledgments

The pages in this volume are not merely the effect of translating words written in a book conceived, and likely already published, in another language. Or maybe they are, but in a very different sense than that entailed by a lighter perspective.[1]

In the words of Antonio Gramsci, translation can be seen as a practice that creates a new product, prompting an endeavor that, even though it refers to another already existing creation – without which it could not exist – develops what has already been postulated in a different light, and precisely in this aspect lies the novelty that enriches the original reflection.

As the mentioned Italian thinker well knew, translation stems from the need to communicate the primary aspect of a discourse, believing it possible, and understanding the emergence of a variation. Thus, the result is always "another" book, another volume that goes beyond the arduous task of finding the most appropriate word, the most accurate term. Even if they have sprung from the same intention, each final version is tied to its own transformations; even more so if, as this version that is introduced in the Anglo-Saxon universe, they include additions and variations contemplating another audience, thinking of other controversies that, even if analog and connected to those of their enunciation context, have their own paths and singularities. For all of these reasons, the translation adds a superlative dignity; it becomes an event enabling a dialogue from the distances and not only in spite of them. From then on, as Jorge Luis Borges would say, what is written belongs less to authors and their obsessions and more to those who consult it with their own concerns. Within this framework, distances fade.

I would like to thank Routledge Publishing House for their trust and support to think about the importance of a particular type of translation – that which refers to psychoanalysis and political theory; to Miño y Dávila Publishing House for facilitating all this process; and to Clara Campero for helping me unveil the nuances of a language that, even if universal, is not my own. I would also like to thank the Gino Germani Institute for Research of the School of Social Sciences of the University of Buenos Aires and all the colleagues researching with tenacity and resolution at this institute, as well as the

National Scientific and Technical Research Council (CONICET, in Spanish), for their support throughout these years, despite political discourses aimed at curbing academic labor based on market demand, always reluctant to reflect on nodal matters such as, for instance, the fascinating fact that we are destined to live together with others.

I thank my friends and colleagues spanning many latitudes who shared their views on the different drafts of this manuscript. To my daughter, Zoe, for embodying not only a responsibility but also hope. And lastly, to my partner, to whom I dedicate this book, given that, for as little as I have been able to express at such dedication in honor of our bond, in times of uncertainty and sadness, there will always remain the beautiful commitment to respect the love and its unexplored corners with the aim of creating, from intimacy, something that may exceed us and be inscribed on another level.

Note

1 *Poderes de la abyección. Política y ontología lacaniana I.* (2021). Buenos Aires: Miño y Dávila.

Foreword

Within our post-colonial and often *crypto-colonial* (Herzfeld, 2002) world, it is not often that one has the opportunity to get in direct contact with dynamic intellectual creation as it unfolds in the so-called Global South. Yet, such encounters can prove extremely beneficial in destabilizing established theoretico-political hierarchies concerning what is primary and what is secondary or utterly insignificant. In a late modern world, in which we often observe supposed "modernity" violently turned upside down, to paraphrase the title of a seminal book by the celebrated English historian Hill (1991), and where the supposed last are often revealed to be first, to use a biblical expression alluding to a rather radical reconstitution of a social hierarchy, the translation and circulation of theoretical production taking place *elsewhere* – in another scene of sorts, with the emphasis not being merely geographical – acquires immense significance.

This is especially the case with Latin America, whose *impure* "semi-periphery" (Mouzelis, 1985) has often experienced first phenomena and patterns that have gone to acquire global relevance.[1] As a result, intellectual output emerging from Latin America obviously deserves to be made available to a global readership and to an international scholarly community that can benefit from the ensuing debate in order to reflect rigorously on shared predicaments. Fortunately, this is already – albeit slowly and rather erratically – happening,[2] and the translation of the work at hand can be seen as belonging to this refreshing wave.

This does not mean, of course, that its significance is to be located outside its own powerful argumentation and its potential scholarly impact, nor that such impetus is emanating from an intellectual space outside (European or euro-centric?) modernity, which can then be used to illuminate what is taking place inside from a radically external – and thus supposedly revelatory – point of view. Of course not. The position from where Laleff Ilieff's argument is articulated is both inside and outside our late modern (potentially universal) politico-philosophical terrain (albeit it shows that the universality at stake can only be a weak, contaminated universality). It is, in other words, *extimate*, in the Lacanian sense of the term. Commanding such an externally intimate vantage point – firmly standing at the threshold – is precisely what allows one to develop an impure yet – by the same token – truly reflexive conceptual and interpretive take on the cruel optimism (Berlant, 2011) of our brutally and violently collapsing and repeatedly reconstituted and (partially) reformulated horizon (both subjective and collective). What allows Ricardo to capture this almost Sisyphean predicament is not, of course, merely geographical location but mainly scholarly effort and intellectual prowess.

Impurity is here an advantage because how else one could positively assess the importance of *negativity*, of what is usually perceived – and thus often marginalized, both in theory and in practice – as a rather disturbing experience destabilizing our sense of order, normality, and identity. As something to be feared, rejected, and tabooed or, at any rate, as something to be controlled; relegated to the "low" and brutish substratum of acceptable – institutionally sanctioned – sociality. Because it is to our conceptualization of the "abject" and "abjection" that this invaluable book is devoted.

It follows Kristeva – who has devoted a whole book on abjection in the 1980s – and through psychoanalysis – focusing on Lacanian (negative) ontology, which already figures prominently in the subtitle – engages in a sustained dialogue with twentieth century and contemporary (mainly political) philosophy: from Bataille, Benjamin, Schmitt, and Girard to Agamben, Clastres, Rancière, Laclau, and Butler. Within this context, and with these main interlocutors, an attempt will be made to encircle metaphorically the traces abjection leaves as the *Real* in politics, which are also crucial in registering its powers. Starting with a challenging discussion of *violence* (which will continue to operate as the spectral backbone of this risky but hugely rewarding journey), Sacrifice, War, and the One will figure, here, as the predominant examples. Without exhausting this debate, they do provide much access to encountering the paradoxical constitution and registering the (circular?) complexity of how something always seems to rely on the violent powers of nothing, with all the instability and impure implications following from such a *Real*-ization (and here, of course, we run the risk of over-simplifying a much more complex and multi-level argument).

Laleff Ilieff heroically assumes the task of addressing head-on the role of the (Lacanian) Real in politics, inclusive of the ultimate (and necessary) failure of such an enterprise, which, of course, does not annul the importance of assuming this task in the first place, in order to illuminate and encircle philosophically and politically the traces it leaves at the intersection between the necessary and the impossible, representation and its limits, order and disorder (violent destruction), power and resistance, as well as the choreography – and the interpenetrations – between them that invariably institute human sociality and political life.

Reading this book, I have personally discovered an intellectual companion and a fellow-traveller sharing similar sensibilities and drawing on common theoretico-political resources of the utmost relevance and promise, locating in a discussion of violence and abjection the *royal road* – a Freudian metaphor, for sure – to encircling the Real in politics, to discussing the *extimate* ambiguity of simultaneously producing/destroying the social order, something crucially relevant to understanding today's paradoxical world.

I am sure the readers of this book will find much that will attract and satisfy them in the standard sense of evaluating a scholarly contribution. Indeed, this is a finely argued, well-grounded, and rich argument of high relevance for assessing contemporary challenges, which *de facto* and dynamically enters into a sustained dialogue with recent interventions highlighting the same conceptual constellation.[3] I also hope that they will also engage with these lines of argumentation present in the text – even in the form of traces of absence or impure formalizations – that are bound to puzzle them, occasionally leading them to (self-)doubts and possibly triggering that paradoxical and painful enjoyment indicating that a true encounter has been made (at the challenging frontier between philosophy and its anti-philosophical beyond).

Yannis Stavrakakis
Professor of Political Discourse Analysis
Aristotle University of Thessaloniki

Notes

1 From the brutal establishment of ordoliberalism in Pinochet's Chile to the contemporary emergence of egalitarian forms of populism against neoliberalism (arguably the so-called Pink Tide prefigured developments in Southern Europe).

2 Of note are publications of the work by established as well as more recently emerging authors such as Dussel, Linera, Palti, and Biglieri and Cadahia.

3 See, for example, Hennefeld and Sammond (2020), and especially the text by Sylvère Lotringer on Bataille and the politics of abjection in the aforementioned collective volume. Bataille is of particular note here, and this is partly acknowledged in Laleff Ilieff's book as well. Responding to the rise of fascism in the 1930s, he was perhaps one of the first to register theoretically the way (sadistic) power structures rely on the isolation and exclusion of the lower classes, which are reduced in this schema to the figure of the abject, "represented from the outside with disgust as the dregs of the people, populace and gutter" (Bataille, 1993, p. 9). Bataille's work is truly illuminating because (1) he captures both the symbolic and significant *affective* aspects of this dehumanizing operation, hence his emphasis on anger, horror, and disgust; (2) bracketing the romantic leftist fantasy that such sadistic operations are automatically met with resistance from the subjects and groups targeted, he thematizes a situation in which abjection is, in fact, eventually accepted and sedimented, leading to political misery, impotence, and resignation (Bataille, 1993, pp. 10–11), perhaps in the intellectual tradition of addressing processes of "voluntary servitude"; (3) he has highlighted how any effective resistance needs to move beyond the intellectual and political elitism and rationalism often plaguing the left and will have to engage with impure political strategies of popular/populist mobilization. Hence his support of Popular Fronts in

the 1930s, a significant example of anti-fascist, egalitarian populism operating from the "low" (Bataille, 1985; also see Stavrakakis, 2024, pp. 35–36). In my recent monograph, *Populist Discourse*: *Recasting Populism Research*, I am briefly discussing Bataille's *base materialism* as a form of materialism consistent with a discursive take on populist politics (Stavrakakis, 2024, pp. 115–118). In my view, a broader assessment of Bataille as a major conceptual and theoretical resource for thinking anew about contemporary politics and populism is still pending and would be extremely beneficial. The same applies to a general discussion of choreographies of abjection in relation to populism. Laleff Ilieff alludes to this connection in the beginning of the fourth part of his book ("The One"), and this may be the place to encourage him to return with a new monograph on this topic!

References

Bataille, G. (1985). Popular front in the street. In G. Bataille (Ed.), *Visions of excess: Selected writings, 1927–1939*, K. R. Lovitt, D. M. Leslie, Jr., & A. Stoekl (Trans. & Eds.), and with an introduction by Allan Stoekl (pp. 161–168). University of Minnesota Press. (Original work published 1935)

Bataille, G. (1993). Abjection and miserable forms. In Y. Shafir (Trans.), Sylvère Lotringer (Ed.), *More & less, vol. 2: Semiotext(e)* (pp. 8–14). (Original work published 1934)

Berlant, L. (2011). *Cruel optimism*. Duke University Press.

Herzfeld, M. (2002). The absent presence: Discourses of crypto-colonialism. *The South-Atlantic Quarterly*, *101*(4), 899–926.

Hennefeld, M., & Sammond, N. (2020). *Abjection incorporated: Mediating the politics of pleasure and violence*. Duke University Press.

Hill, C. (1991). *The world turned upside down: Radical ideas during the English revolution*. Penguin.

Mouzelis, N. (1985). *Politics in the semi-periphery: Early parliamentarism and late industrialisation in the Balkans and Latin America*. Palgrave-Macmillan.

Stavrakakis, Y. (2024). *Populist discourse: Recasting populism research*. Routledge.

Introduction

To conceive of the Real [*réel*] as impossible does not mean that we cannot attempt to make the impossible the object of certain reflections. Time and again, we merely talk about the challenge of the power of words. So it is that we find ourselves already pervaded by impossibility. As Jacques Lacan would argue, the truth is expressed as "half-saying". This means that any saying that is overwhelmed or insufficient is always already impossible.[1] However, it is precisely because of this that one cannot ignore the status of the Real, which is no more than a representation of a slice of existence. We are condemned to the Real, and not because the Real is a form of the absolute, one that transcends any symbolic inscription and grounds it from an outside; nor is it because the Real is a mere limitation or *tyché*. Put simply, between the vision of a pure and pristine event and one that establishes the possibilities of a full symbolization, it is necessary to establish a different notion of the Real, one that forces us to consider the ontology that operates behind the discourses, especially the discourses on politics.

My intention in this book is precisely to consider the Real in politics. To do so, I will use the category of abjection. I will attempt to analyze how "something" appears where nothing should appear, and in doing so, examine the assumptions and limits of community life and the circumstances of its structuring. The abject, then, shall be understood as a disturbing expression that is located – without blocking it or denying it, but rather alluding to it – in the gap [*béance*] of existence. I will look at certain conceptual ideas concerning the instituting dimension and the always contingent articulations that continuously surface in social life, with a view to reflecting on what constitutes the instability of a space of representation and its new findings that seek to solve that representation. I will argue that abjection is something more than a theme adjacent to the variations, rectifications, and modulations that any order attempts in its ever-dynamic search to capture what emerges and to grasp what might disrupt it by expressing the impossibility of a definitive stabilization. The abject will not, therefore, be judged as an expression that operates on the margins of the social, or as that which comes from inversion, or from the knowledge of an excluded other; rather, it shall be represented as the point where the failure of

DOI: 10.4324/9781003457022-1

any identity is revealed, the point of non-sense that enables the political and these other subsequent operations.[2] This will permit me to show that any full apprehension by the symbolic is, from the outset, an illusion; something will always remain impossible to assimilate, as a remainder and not as a slag of significance,[3] and it is on this aspect that I intend to focus.

Politics unfolds from an ineradicable hole. I will take some figures that pervade certain contemporary discourses to show this, and as a kind of effect inherent to this interpretative movement, I will observe a certain real dimension in the theory, a dimension that makes the metaphorical and non-conceptuality (Blumenberg, 1997).[4] Far from being an exercise in denunciation, this work sets out to question assumptions and perspectives present in different approaches to politics; approaches that inform or show how abjection should (not) be understood. If in doing so I use Lacan's words, it is because I consider that they offer us an improved understanding of these aspects.

Throughout his teachings, Lacan showed that the knotting between the registers of the Real, the Symbolic, and the Imaginary gives support to a reality whose void cannot be filled, merely precariously covered over; hence, from Lacan's perspective, the only reality is an interlacing of the strings. For this reason, the Borromean knot "has a definitive property: it suffices for one of the three loops it knots together to fall away for all the others to disperse" (Milner, 2021, p. 91).[5]

Having said this, my motivation is clearly part of the tradition of political theory, while my starting point is none other than the ontological coordinates advocated by Lacanian psychoanalysis. I am aware that an exercise such as this, which uses a cross-disciplinary approach, should be undertaken with some

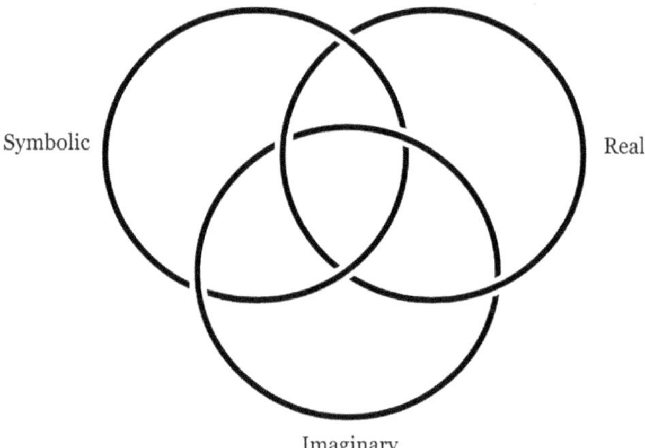

Figure 0.1 The Borromean knot

precaution. Although this is not a pioneering endeavor, mobilizing politics and psychoanalysis calls for the ever-novel act of clearly stating the premises delimiting the proposed reflection. First of all, it is important to point out that this is not an essay in favor of some sort of complementarity. To be quite clear, between politics and psychoanalysis "there's no such thing as a sexual relationship" [*il n'y a pas de rapport sexuel*]; between politics and psychoanalysis there is a logic of the reverse [*l'envers*] (Lacan, 2007), which understands specificities and often contradictory dynamics, where the complexity of the frameworks of meaning stands out.[6]

There is no denying that politics operates in the field of identifications, while psychoanalysis, in its journey through the tribulations of desire, tends to make its review by questioning imperatives, highlighting the signifiers that mark an age and cause unrest, and which inevitably bind subjects to their time. For this reason, I recommend sparing use of what appears when both logics come into play. To consider politics using concepts of psychoanalysis allows us to deal with things that often appear as mere background noise, whose indistinguishable appearance challenges any definition. That whisper – which is not the Real but which expresses it as a weakness of the imposed voice – will be judged as an echo of the lack [*manque*] and thus as a feature that allows us to doubt the field of politics itself. In this sense, I will focus on the field that Ernesto Laclau noted when he defined the matter on which his own research was based:

> So, the crucial task is to think the specificity of discursive formations in such terms that the interaction between the various instances and registers loses its purely casual and external character and becomes constitutive of the instances themselves. This clearly requires a new ontology. I see the psychoanalytic revolution as an immense widening of the field of objectivity, bringing to consideration kinds of relations between entities which cannot be grasped with the conceptual arsenal of classical ontology. I see as our main intellectual task to rethink philosophy in the light of this project.
>
> (Laclau, 2004, p. 304)[7]

However, unlike Laclau's work, which sought to specify the dynamics of forging collective identities with their discourse shifts, their overdeterminations and equivalences, mine shall be much more modest and limited in its scope: I will attempt to explain certain elements that operate on the very basis of the social; I will try to consider politics from an ontological perspective, rooted in Lacanian theory, which can well be considered "negative" (Stavrakakis, 2000) since it feeds on the lack of a substrate of truth and the impossibilities of every decision. Or, in other words, from a "non-ontology", since, according to Lacan himself, nothing can be ascertained about the being since the being does not exist; it lacks substance. Having said this, how is it possible to suggest an anti-ontological thinking on ontology? The answer does not entail a diversion maneuver or a shortcut, only a clarification.

For this purpose, I refer to Alfredo Eidelsztein (2009), who in his attempt to show *another* Lacan – one far removed from the core aspects put forward by his son-in-law and trustee Jacques-Alain Miller – highlights the difference that Lacan introduced in relation to Freud.

Eidelsztein argues that there is less of a continuity than a separation between Freud and Lacan – a hiatus. While Freud developed his considerations based on a view influenced by biologicist discourse – a view that would lead him to show the body as a scenario for drive – Lacan merely translated to clinical practice a view that prevents the assertion of a truth that is no longer the field of the Symbolic and, therefore, is a non-truth or a half-truth. So from Lacan's perspective, drive would always be imbued with the Symbolic.[8] Therefore, from a reading of Eidelsztein, thinking *le retour à* Freud suggested by Eidelsztein at the beginning of his seminar was imposed as part of a reaffirmation of Freud's words; in this reading, he may have introduced some important developments on the Freudian path. However, in reviewing the different meanings of the term in French, Eidelsztein claims that Lacan proposed a kind of journey, a veritable return intended to stir up Freud. So Lacan would have then made not so much a rectification as a genuine renewal of psychoanalysis and its clinical guidelines.

As can be deduced from this, Eidelsztein's reading goes against Miller, who tends to distinguish different periods in Lacan's teachings, seeking to first see a Lacan of the "Imaginary", then a Lacan of the "Symbolic", and finally one "last" Lacan focused on the "Real", as if this were actually possible. According to Eidelsztein, Miller makes a mistake that is not only epistemological, since what he postulates is an equivalence between the Real and the body based on the notion of *jouissance*, which modifies the direction of the cure. Thus, Miller would suggest an erroneous conception of the knot, favoring one register over the idea of the knotting. Consequently, Eidelsztein says, Lacanians merely reactivate, more or less surreptitiously, the biologicism present in Freud, which is what Lacan sought to abandon definitively. As we shall see in the following chapter, this appears to be a debt imposed more by Lacan's followers than by his work – a debt that condemns *jouissance* to a pre-symbolic, natural dimension that each individual would possess.[9] Following this idea, clinical practice should be oriented toward elucidating a particular way of doing with *jouissance* – a way of doing that is always isolated – renouncing thinking about the effect of the Other and their discourses on the subject, their sufferings, and their identifications. Eidelsztein writes that the effect borders on individualism or, if one prefers, nihilism, a perspective that removes the individual from the social.[10]

What is interesting about Eidelsztein's reading is that he argues that the logic of the knotting prevails over the relevance of each register, emphasizing what I will explore in Chapter 2, namely, the impossibility of thinking the political by divorcing the registers, since otherwise we would be pinning down a point of analysis and ignoring the complexity of the framework that constitutes social life. It is useful here to recall Alenka Zupančič's ideas to be even clearer on this aspect.

Zupančič's interesting study puts forward a more complex dimension in Lacan that goes far beyond the prevailing atomistic logic in the sphere of clinical practice and the subjectivity of our era. Zupančič argues that the Symbolic is always operating, so it cannot be ignored when considering *jouissance*, nor in the unease implied in its satisfaction. Indeed, she writes that

> there is no natural need that would be absolutely pure, i.e. devoid of this surplus element which splits it from within. This split, this interval or void, this original non-convergence of two different versants of the satisfaction is, for Freud, the very site or ground of human sexuality.
>
> (Zupančič, 2008: 9)

Unlike Eidelsztein, Zupančič does not find a trace of biologicism in the Freudian notion of libido, quite the contrary:

> If Freud uses the term 'libido' to refer to a certain field of 'energy', it is to refer to it as a surplus energy, and not to any kind of general energetic level involved in our lives. It cannot designate the whole of energy (as Jung suggested).
>
> (2008: 10)

Zupančič goes as far as to claim that the sexual is a "concept of a radical ontological impasse" (2008, p. 16), which may bring to mind the Lacanian variation since it is this impasse that, when formulating a notion such as *object a* – that is, the object that alludes to the lack of object – underlines what Freud did not thematize or thematized differently by assuming the existence of a grounds, a real substratum. However, aside from the debate on the spirit that brings the Freudian work alive – which I do not intend to settle here, only indicate for the purposes of thinking about the different perspectives in the way the political is conceived – in Zupančič's opinion in the notion of libido, it seems that the ontological displacement that Lacan undertakes from the Borromean knot is already operating. Consequently, it is evident that Zupančič reads Freud based on Lacan without realizing the difference I note here.

As I said, Lacan adopted an anti-ontological stance throughout his teachings; in fact, he mocked ontology in several seminars. This can be seen in his invention of two neologisms: *hontologie* (Lacan, 1998, 2007) – a clear pun of the French terms *ontologie* and *honte*, meaning "shame" – and *ontotautologie* (Lacan, 2018), which refers to the term "tautology". As Milner and Alain Badiou note, this should be included in the context of an "anti-philosophical" perspective. What do I mean by this?

Badiou (2018) argues that Lacan was an anti-philosopher in attempting to establish a view opposing traditional metaphysics – a tradition which, incidentally, he revisited constantly – seeking to make a break with some of its assumptions. In particular, he criticized both philosophers' inclination to assert the impossible as possible and psychoanalysts' tendency to refuse to measure themselves against other discourses. Lacan pointed out to philosophers the impossibility of a saying about the truth, stressing their shortcoming in being unable to specify the status of the Real, while to psychoanalysts – his students and colleagues – he pointed out the need to correctly situate which epistemological premises should guide analytical practice. In this context, he used mathematics – especially the formulation of mathemes – to illustrate the problem of truth, which is none other, in his opinion, than properly circumscribing the insistence of the Real to be inscribed in the absence of meaning and ultimate affirmation – that is, the very hole of the Symbolic. Thus, in Lacan's view, "truth" and "meaning" are only knotted together by the action of knowing, an action that is an operation that plugs the void, as philosophy has done and, as Heidegger said, as theology did before, since both discourses have sought to postulate themselves as embodiments of the "master's discourse".[11]

Lacan's anti-philosophical stance explains his conviction about the "non-being". Lacan believed that not only is there no truth but also there is no subject who can rediscover it, much less from an intimate or hidden core of meaning. It is here that Eidelsztein's position becomes particularly interesting for this study. The "lack-of-being" [*manque à être*] is the beacon that indicates the impossibility of reducing *jouissance* to a natural, bodily, or biological element. *Jouissance* must be understood as an indication that there exists a saying that is prior to the subject, in which the subject is uniquely inscribed and on which it does not cease to operate. Thus, the "lack-of-being" explains that the being is without essence; it is a being of the lack; it only is by existing and being. Hence, the Symbolic – the law, the word, the signifier – does not intervene by cutting a natural substance; it does not operate by suppressing something already given. This is not Freud's famous Oedipus trauma. For Lacan, there is nothing that existed first; hence, all his clinical conception revolves around the *parlêtre* – a neologism formed from *parler*, "to speak", and *être*, "to be" – and not around the being or the soul. Herein lies his distance from classical philosophy and ontology! That said, we understand why *jouissance* is not the Real that circulates in the biological body and appears as a symptom because of the intervention of the social; it is an always symbolic dimension that reveals the lack of meaning and, hence, a complex relationship with the Real.[12] Depending on how the knotting of registers is conceived, not only a specific kind of clinical practice emerges, but also – and this is what interests me – there also emerges a way of reading politics, its conflicts and constitutive disagreements, its interventions and administrations.

For these reasons, I argue that although Lacan opposed ontology because of his concern for the being, his denunciation and disagreement led him to postulate a new perspective on ontology, which can be deemed a "negative" ontology or a "non-ontology". And this stems precisely from his anti-philosophical stance.

It is important to note here that when analyzing the gap of social life through the abject, it is possible to observe the attempts to close it and to manage it by politicizing and depoliticizing instances, mechanisms inherent to politics.[13] It is possible to note the real nature of every symbolic order and its capacity to give an identity to the space of representation, and it can even be considered that every identity has an imaginary dimension as support, which enables the knotting between the Symbolic and the Real.[14] What I want to highlight here is that the abject indicates how every definition or frontier, necessary for the social bond, retains a non-meaning; hence its intrinsic metaphorical dimension, since it always alludes to something else that is not said, that cannot be entirely said, because it never is, except as history.

The notion of "extimacy" [*extimité*] is essential here. This neologism, which Lacan coined and used only once in his seminar VII, *The Ethics of Psychoanalysis* [1959–1960], shows how the symbolic lacks guarantees and is articulated by exceeding the subject itself. Miller (1988) has analyzed it most accurately in pointing out its construction from the term "intimacy", which means it is not to be understood in the play of opposites. In fact, Miller argues that "extimacy" seeks to explain the intimate, even the most intimate, based on what seems to be the external or foreign. Thus, if the most intimate is on the outside and everything in that domain appears as a foreign body, this means that symbolic imperatives cannot be understood as distance or imposition but as an example of articulation between the singular dimension and the collective dimension, since the subject is only in the social sphere.[15] This is probably easier to grasp by following the example that Miller offers with the Augustinian expression that references God as "*interior intimo meo*, 'more interior than my innermost being'" (1988, p. 123). Thus, the place that Augustine of Hippo assigned to the Creator is, in the field of psychoanalysis, the place of the Other:

> Which other is this, then, to whom I am more attached than to myself [*moi*], since, at the most assented to heart of my identity to myself, he pulls the strings?
>
> His presence can only be understood in an alterity raised to the second power, which already situates him in a mediating position in relation to my own splitting from myself, as if from a semblable.
>
> (Lacan, 2006b: 436)

In short, extimacy shows how the law is introjected at the same time that, because of that movement, the lack of substance is shown, the impossibility of resorting to a substrate of the being. The "Big Other", therefore, does not exist; it is perforated: "There is no Other of the Other". In any case, the ordering dimension of the Symbolic implies that function that Lacan called "The Name-of-the-Father", that is, the fundamental metaphor that functions as a nodal point [*point de capiton*] between signifier and sense. As we will see here, there is a suggestion that this is a function as necessary as it is impossible.

The lack, present in the subject itself, is also a lack in the social order. If, in order to become a subject, the human cub must surrender a "pound of flesh" (Lacan, 2014, p. 124) to signification, this is only articulated with the very lack of signification that makes the paternal, regulatory metaphor necessary. Freud expressed this in part in *Civilization and Its Discontents* [1930], which Lacan took up with renewed vim, speaking of "symbolic castration", that is, a cut that shows the impossibility of the whole and the non-whole that works in the very interior of order.[16]

For this reason, it can be said that abjection is connected with this structural aspect and consequently crosses through politics. So it is that this book sets out to consider the hiatus at the heart of identity – a hiatus that goes beyond the figure of a "constitutive outside" or of an other from which recognition is formed. In Lacanian non-ontology, there is no dialectics possible, even in spite of the ingenious arguments of Žižek (2013), who always tends to see the remainder and not the closure in the Hegelian movement, a matter which, in his opinion, Lacan would have grasped well.[17] The abject, I repeat, is not only what appears displaced by the social order; if anything, it is what should be displaced because it alludes to the void of the social, to the problem of any decision, but which can never be structurally eliminated, only precariously pursued.

To better clarify the meaning I intend for this concept, I will outline here the path I propose. In the first chapter, I will give a brief overview to show the course of the notion, though without aiming to carry out a genealogy in the strict sense. Rather, I will show the connection between abjection and Freud's formulations on the Uncanny [*Das Unheimliche*] to then see the shift that Lacan's reading makes, precisely from ontology. This will enable me to refer to the explicit treatment by Georges Bataille and Judith Butler. However, I will explore one point, especially a kind of middle ground between these two authors, for it was Julia Kristeva who decisively recovered this category in *Powers of Horror: An Essay on Abjection* [1980]. I consider this essay a most valuable precedent to my own interpretative work. In my view, Kristeva thoroughly shows – albeit not down to the ultimate consequences – how the abject is a kind of Real that operates from within and not only from outside of the Symbolic. This overview will allow me to reinforce the dimension of extimacy in all identity, as I have suggested earlier. However, unlike that of Bataille, Kristeva, or Butler, my approach needs strengthening or an additional thematization that can adequately situate the abject in the non-ontological territory. This is primarily due to the fact that abjection cannot suggest an unknotting of the three registers of experience – Real, Symbolic, and Imaginary; on the contrary, it reaffirms what the knot is meant to saturate. However, as we shall see, some theoretical discourses tend to absolutize one of these, ignoring their political effects and weakening the very understanding of the political. I will thus aim to express a kind of distinction to illustrate why we should not give more importance to one dimension over another. Only this way will we understand something about the Real in politics.

Following this question, in the second chapter, I will review Walter Benjamin's celebrated "Toward the Critique of Violence" [1921]. I will read Benjamin's arguments as a way of rejecting the Symbolic. I will argue that, in this essay at least, Benjamin renounces thinking the political as such, as he formulates not a pre-symbolic instance – as can be read in Kristeva – or an element subsumed *in* the Symbolic – as can be found in Butler – but rather a "pure Real", which annuls the Symbolic and which cannot assume the tragedy of politics, that is, a world without guarantees, an unfinished, always contingent action.[18]

The three following parts offer an analysis of abjection that will reinstate specific figures or metaphors that explain abjection, allude to it, and show its aspects. I concentrate specifically on three aspects – Sacrifice, War, and the One – in the knowledge that I will be far from exhausting the subject, let alone considering other interesting, connected instances that shed light on the tribulations of sovereignty, the State, and community order in Modernity. With this accepted limit, I will embark on the challenge of thinking about various authors such as René Girard, Giorgio Agamben, Carl Schmitt, Pierre Clastres, and Jacques Rancière, who have laid invaluable foundations for me to express *something* about the Real in politics from the perspective of abjection.

Notes

1 "It is very clear also that I am not talking about everything. It is even in what I state, it resists anyone saying everything about it. You can put your finger on that every day. Even on the fact that I state that I am not saying everything, that is something different, as I already said, that comes from the fact that the truth is only a half-saying" (Lacan, 1971, no page number).

2 This implies that, in ontic terms, the abject may appear in different ways; it may be symbolized in various ways. My emphasis, then, is on understanding how its emergence is conceived and how it operates in its assumptions and perspectives.

3 In Lacan's words, "In human destiny, the remainder is always fruitful. The slag is the extinguished remainder" (1998, p. 134).

4 The theoretical gap that makes it possible to inform the Real in politics has a historical field that enables it. Palti (2017) describes it very well in his accurate work of historical-conceptual reconstruction. Although the approach adopted here is different from Palti's, I certainly take many of his arguments as a reference framework, and I share many of his conclusions.

5 For the purposes of orientation, it could be said – simplifying a little – that the understanding of the Real as the impossible means conceiving of the Symbolic from the register of the signifier, from the actions of the structure, that is, from the formation of an order that is nothing without its flaws, and the Imaginary as a register that appeals to the image [*imago*], to such perceptions and representations that separate and unite, that divide and suture, a field of representation. As we will see, this imaginary support becomes crucial in considering abjection. Recall that in his seminar on anxiety,

Lacan (2014) understood that the process of formation of the subject entails the production of a remainder that is impossible to assimilate – the *object a* – that is, a Real that cannot be absorbed by symbolization – something radically heterogeneous, in the words of Laclau (2005) – which functions as a cause of desire or surplus-jouissance [*plus-de-jouir*]. The *object a* is located, precisely, at the center of the knot, that is, in the place of the lack. As discussed below, the abject is connected with the semblant; it goes no longer against the norm but as an expression of the abnormal character of any norm. For further reading on registers, I recommend Jameson's classic work (1977). On the introduction of the Borromean knot in Lacan's work, see Roudinesco (1997). On its importance and its use in considering current politics, see, among other sources, Alemán (2024).

6 It is no coincidence that the crossover between social sciences and psychoanalysis – as Lacan's own history shows – is highly productive. On this matter, see Parker and Pavón-Cuéllar (2021), Zafiropoulos (2001), and the thought-provoking writings of Stavrakakis (2000, 2007, 2020).

7 Stavrakakis makes an interesting point on Laclau's relationship with psychoanalysis: "To be sure, Laclau's work has been crucial in developing the social and political relevance both of Lacanian constructionism and of Lacan's negative ontology. His work has been paradigmatic in simultaneously highlighting the political workings of the symbolic and in registering the real limits of signification. However, this should not be interpreted as a sign of limitless convergence or fusion between Laclau and Lacanian theory" (2007, p. 19). In this line, I consider it possible to read Laclau with Lacan, in spite of, in many places, Laclau's own structuralist resistances.

8 "I ought to warn you: the 'apparatus of the body' does not match the biological body. In other words, the drive is regarding the instinct, what the body as apparatus is regarding the biological body. An apparatus is an artificial instrument that involves a set of parts or system. And if Lacan states that something is structured in the same way, that is because the apparatus of the body is a system of parts with gaps, like the ones we find in the networks of signifiers" (Eidelsztein, 2009, p. 212).

9 "To sum up: the sexual drive only represents sexuality within psychic life; it does not represent the biological body. Because the drive 'represents', we are immediately led to the field of the signifier. This is why the drive has the structure of a montage: it shows the solidarity with the montage that the net of signifiers imposes on it" (Eidelsztein, 2009, p. 209).

10 However, it is not entirely clear what the orientation of the clinical practice would be for Eidelsztein, since, at times, it might seem that he suggests enabling processes of identification-unidentification, which, of course, cannot be detached from the Other. This might very interestingly indicate that the cure implies a political edge, but we still need to think about the dimension of singularity in the manner in which we conceive the Symbolic.

11 Heidegger argues that theology does not assume the void by always postulating God as the answer: "The heaviest blow against God is not that God is held to be unknowable, not that God's existence is demonstrated to be unprovable, but rather that the god held to be real is elevated to the highest value. For this blow comes precisely not from those who are standing about,

who do not believe in God, but from the believers and their theologians who discourse in the being that is of all beings most in being, without ever letting it occur to them to think on Being itself, in order thereby to become aware that, seen from out of faith, their thinking and their talking is sheer blasphemy if it meddles in the theology of faith" (1977, p. 105).

12 Indeed, in Néstor Braunstein's book (2021) on the notion of *jouissance* – probably the book that has shed the most light on the subject to date – the Real is represented with some ambivalence, that is, at times tied to the pre-symbolic of the *jouissance* of the body, at times inscribed in the symbolization in which the body necessarily appears inserted. Note the following extract: "Nothing remains from an original *jouissance* but the nostalgia that creates and mythologizes it retroactively, beginning with the fact that it has been lost, is irrecoverable in its 'original' form, and must be veered through other means, perverted. The body, an unlimited reservoir of *jouissance* in principle, is progressively emptied of that substance (mythical libidinal fluid) that moved through its pores, flooded its recesses, and settled in the borders of its orifices. Now it can be reached, yes, but only through the detour of narcissism, the field of images and words, as a *langagière jouissance*, outside the body (*hors corps*), subject to the imperatives and aspirations of the ideal ego that commands them with the false promise of its recovery in the ego ideal [I(A)]" (2020, p. 51). For these reasons, I consider it risky to sustain the fiction of self-ownership of the body, making it the point of attack of a political view.

13 In my previous book, I studied the dynamics between politicization and de-politicization (Laleff Ilieff, 2020). In this context, I dialogued with the ideas of Kalyvas (2000).

14 I follow the indication that Lacan made in his unpublished seminar titled *RSI* (1974–1975).

15 This brings us back to the problem of clinical practice mentioned earlier. However, this is not a psychoanalytical clinical exercise but a theoretical-political reflection using psychoanalysis.

16 This is not to be confused with the idea of sacrifice. There is no sacrifice in the entry to symbolization. The decision is unfathomable; sacrifice can only be read retroactively as a loss of what was never had, that is, as a symbolic dimension. This distinction is crucial: In Freud's view, the natural bond with the mother is lost, and it is a question of its mnemic trace; in Lacan's, it is about the experience of the lack of that which never existed and its possibility of positivizing lack in desire.

17 This influence is also found in works such as McGowan's (2019). The problem with Žižek is that he tends to read Hegel from a Lacanian perspective and Lacan from a Hegelian perspective, without showing that this is the distinctive sign of his own theoretical operation and not the permanence of a single framework of intelligibility that invariably goes from Hegel to Lacan.

18 I should clarify here that precisely because of contingency, political action is historical; therefore, not all the imaginable political possibilities are possible, only those that can do something with a frame of reference and that find grounds to be legitimate.

Part One

The Real and the Symbolic

1 The Uncanny

Freud's short 1919 essay "The Uncanny" [*Das Unheimliche*] contains a fundamental aspect that sheds light on what is encapsulated in the notion of abjection.

In this text, Freud speaks of a component that operates in some expressions of anxiety. He notes that it is something linked with the abominable or the despicable that appears as a threat but nonetheless comes from somewhere intimate. To better clarify this issue, from the first lines, Freud seeks to clarify the field of inquiry. He says that he does not intend to explore aesthetics, a discipline that deals "with what is beautiful, attractive and sublime – that is, with feelings of a positive nature – and with the circumstances and the objects that call them forth, rather than with the opposite feelings of repulsion and distress" (1981, p. 219),[1] nor does he intend to refer to an ethical matter. He says that his goal is purely clinical, while still noting the two possible paths of his inquiry; both, however, lead to the same place: The uncanny refers to something as intimate and familiar as it is distant.

> Two courses are open to us at the outset. Either we can find out what meaning has come to be attached to the word "uncanny" in the course of its history; or we can collect all those properties of persons, things, sense-impressions, experiences and situations which arouse in us the feeling of uncanniness, and then infer the unknown nature of the uncanny from what all these examples have in common. I will say at once that both courses lead to the same result: the uncanny is that class of the frightening which leads back to what is known of old and long familiar. How this is possible, in what circumstances the familiar can become uncanny and frightening, I shall show in what follows. Let me also add that my investigation was actually begun by collecting a number of individual cases, and was only later confirmed by an examination of linguistic usage. In this discussion, however, I shall follow the reverse course.
>
> (1981, p. 220)

In order to justify this evaluation, Freud begins with a philological analysis over a few pages. He notes that it is "the opposite of *heimlich* ['homely'],

DOI: 10.4324/9781003457022-3

heimisch ['native'] – the opposite of what is familiar; and we are tempted to conclude that what is 'uncanny' is frightening precisely because it is not known and familiar". However, he claims that not everything new and unfamiliar is frightening; "something has to be added to what is novel and unfamiliar in order to make it uncanny" (1981, p. 220). This, he says, is something that Ernst Jentsch did not grasp; his research into psychiatry did not go beyond noting the connection between the uncanny and the novel. After reviewing translations of the uncanny in different languages – such as Latin, Greek, English, French, and Spanish – Freud returns to his mother tongue to observe that, despite its multiple meanings, "the word '*heimlich*' exhibits one which is identical with its opposite, '*unheimlich*'. What is *heimlich* thus comes to be *unheimlich*" (1981, p. 224). Here he notes that it was Friedrich Schelling, the famous German philosopher, who wrote something entirely new and unpredicted:

> Thus, *heimlich* is a word the meaning of which develops in the direction of ambivalence, until it finally coincides with its opposite, *unheimlich. Unheimlich* is in some way or other a sub-species of *heimlich*. Let us bear this discovery in mind, though we cannot yet rightly understand it, alongside of Schelling's definition of the *Unheimlich*. If we go on to examine individual instances of uncanniness, these hints will become intelligible to us.
>
> (1981, p. 226)

Freud endorses Schelling's assessment by referring to the Brothers Grimm dictionaries, in which the term *unheimlich* appears as a variant of *heimlich*. He explores this ambivalence later on by returning to some stories and tales. He mainly refers to "The Sandman", written by another Romantic author, ETA Hoffmann – whom he considers the "unrivalled master of the uncanny in literature" (1981, p. 233) – to argue that the *unheimlich* refers to his protagonists' distressing experiences due to an element considered terrifying, likely referring back to some childhood experience. Thus, it is present in the fear of organ mutilation, in the representation of a double that torments identity – as in "The Sand-Man" – and in other terrifying fantasies that occupy, Freud argues, a major role in the spiritual life of neurotics, due to the anxiety of "the castration complex of childhood" (1981, p. 233) and the "constant recurrence of the same thing" (1981, p. 234), which could well be due to the critical instances of the "ego", which are found in the initial stages of narcissism. Consequently, the remarkable nature of cases in which the uncanny is manifested reaffirms its value in the structural processes that give life to subjects' psyches.

Freud thus shows that the uncanny threatens the identity, destabilizing it; it appears as external to it when, in fact, it constitutes it from within. So it is that Milner writes that "the unheimlich is not the inverse of the familiar, but something familiar infected with an anxiety that shatters it" (2021, p. 43), since there is a frontier between the intimate and the foreign, between the "ego" and its surrounding world, which, far from being impassable, shows how unstable every determination is – which leads again to extimacy.[2]

But the issue here is that the Freudian uncanny suggests an idea of return. On this point, Freud's perspective seems to be in agreement with Lacan's first definition, understanding the Real as that which "always returns to the same place" (2019, p. 480), as he said in seminar VI, *Desire and Its Interpretation* [1958–1959]. However, intricate theoretical perspectives can be derived from this definition of the Real. Thus, I believe it is crucial in this first chapter to discern how the Freudian uncanny is tied to this problematic idea of the Real as return that demands the circumscription of the abject in a different manner, that is, in a non-ontology that starts from the necessary and contingent knotting of the three registers.

To simply postulate the idea of "return of the Real" may suggest a certain prevalence of the Real over the Symbolic and the Imaginary, a prevalence that I deem erroneous and unhelpful. It may even suggest that the Real existed first and then the other two registers came, ignoring the covariant nature that it instills in Lacan's negative ontology. Otherwise, it would be a component that was captured by the knot, but that existed before it and outside of it and still exists as a trace. That is, it would be to suggest that the Real was at some point "pure", something independent from the Symbolic and the Imaginary and which, for that reason, persists as a trace in the symbolization or as nature that symbolization comes to dominate or prevail over. However, the Real, displaced by repression or symbolic castration, would always manage to realize itself and fulfill a kind of destiny. This too would give weight to an idea that locates politics in that pre-symbolic element, as a source of resistance or as an equivalence that assumes the "natural" with a meaning. I believe that this was not the meaning that Lacan intended, and consequently he then changed his definition. To fully understand this matter, I propose to identify the central points of Lacan's reading of "The Uncanny", as it is precisely here that a shift occurs that is essential for my theoretical-political reflection.[3]

In his seminar on anxiety in 1962–1963, Lacan associates the *unheimlich* with the figure of the big Other, noting the scant attention given to Freud's essay. He says it is:

> [an] article that I've never heard anyone comment on and no one seems to have noticed that it's indispensable for broaching the question of anxiety. Just as I broached the unconscious with the *Witz*, this year I'm going to be broaching anxiety with the *Unheimliche*.
>
> (2014, p. 41)

He also notes that

> the *Unheimliche* is what appears at the place where the minus-*phi* should be. Indeed, everything starts with imaginary castration, because there is no

> image of lack, and with good reason. When something does appear there, it is, therefore, if I may put it this way, because lack happens to be lacking.
>
> (2014, p. 41)

Consequently, Lacan connects the Freudian uncanny with his ideas on the specular dimension of the "Mirror Stage" (Lacan, 2006c), ideas that indicate the support that the Other gives in the evolution of the subject. The uncanny would then serve to reveal the lack and its shift from the field of identity, since its place is the site of an impossible remainder that threatens image unity. This nonetheless shows a paradox: Where nothing should appear, something emerges and haunts the integrity of the subject. This image indicates that something is lacking, and that what is lacking is none other than the lack of the image that the Other generates. Consequently, Lacan indicates that anxiety presents itself in that same place and is linked to the object, the small object *a*, which by definition is impossible to symbolize; hence, this is not anxiety over a loss, but anxiety over a structural lack, for its demonstration, for the hollow nature of the Symbolic. As Zupančič writes, "His claim is that at the bottom of anxiety, there is not a (revived) fear or menace of castration", but "a fear or menace of losing the castration itself, that is to say, of losing the symbolic support provided by the castration complex" (2008, p. 52).

This Lacanian reading of the Freudian *Unheimliche* carries with it the redefinition of castration: The Other has no guarantees; the Other cannot answer for that image; the Other does not exist. Lacan rightly understood this problem as necessarily linked with the path of desire. For these reasons, he showed the role of fantasy [*fantasme*], which obstructs the constitutive gap:

> At this point *Heim*, what shows itself isn't simply what you've always known, that desire reveals itself as desire of the Other, here desire in the Other, but also that my desire, I shall say, enters the lair where it has been awaited for all eternity in the shape of the object that I am in so far as it exiles me from my subjectivity, by deciding on its own all the signifiers to which this subjectivity is attached.
>
> (Lacan, 2014, p. 48)

This Lacanian reading of the Freudian uncanny reveals the very lack of the Symbolic, the scarcity that is not of the object but of the being itself. This serves to understand the abject less as the name of that lack and more as the impossible name that appears because of that lack: i.e. the uncanny image of an identity that is intrinsically dislocated, without accepting the failure of every norm, its incapacity.

I will now associate Lacan's crucial resignification of the *unheimliche* with the term abjection, identifying what I deem to be the fundamental aspects that allow us to specifically explain certain theoretical-political problems from the perspective of Lacanian ontology. I will begin with an essay by Georges

Bataille, titled "Abjection and Miserable Forms" [1934], in which he shows the imperative act of exclusion that constitutes the grounds for collective existence.

In Bataille's view (1993), abjection is a process that marks the impotence of the displaced, its oppression, which is different from the sexual perversions in which abject things are sought. Abjection relegates subjects with the aim of blocking their own capacity to effectuate the act of exclusion that defines them. And although Bataille says that this process is the work of all men and women, he notes that, like the many victims of physical or mental illnesses, in the contemporary world the majority are incapable of reacting strongly against the rot that invades them. It is because of this oppression that life is situated under the humane level. In Bataille's view, abjection entails a dimension that derives from the substantial incapacity to avoid contact with abject things, which is essentially the abjection of things communicated to the men that touch them.[4]

In short, Bataille argues that it is not a question of men and women being enshrined as beings of abjection but of turning them into its targets, which reduces their capacity for executing a subversion that reshapes the frontiers of the social.[5]

Kristeva, in *Powers of Horror*, also sees abjection as a phenomenon linked with exclusions. From her perspective, it is a dimension belonging to the social and symbolic order that is displaced at both individual and social levels. Kristeva argues that the abject is more violent than the Freudian uncanny: "Essentially different from 'uncanniness', more violent, too, abjection is elaborated through a failure to recognize its kin; nothing is familiar, not even the shadow of a memory" (1982, p. 5).

It is important to note this difference that Kristeva points out in Freud's conceptualization. In her words, "all abjection is in fact recognition of the want on which any being, meaning, language, or desire is founded" (1982, p. 5). With a similar statement, the author seemingly intends to observe the eminently ontological dimension that shows the impossibility of fixing an ultimate meaning on social life: "The experience of *want* itself as logically preliminary to being and object – to the being of the object" (1982, p. 5). Indeed, Kristeva stressed that the abject denotes the non-sense of all sense and the need to exclude that which threatens order, that which is radically heterogeneous.

However, moving away from Bataille's subject-object and Freud's familiar-unfamiliar distinctions, Kristeva notes that abjection has an unintentionally perverse dimension in that it does not abandon or assume an interdiction, a rule, or a law, but rather deviates it and corrupts it. From this perspective, the abject cannot be blocked but is only seen in its traumatic emergences – as Freud said – since it is always present and appeals where meaning collapses. Kristeva argues that this explains why it threatens even though its location, its place of birth, cannot be distinguished: "There looms, within abjection, one of those violent, dark revolts of being, directed against a threat that seems to emanate from an exorbitant outside or inside, ejected beyond the scope of the possible, the tolerable, the thinkable. It lies there, quite close, but it cannot be assimilated" (1982, p. 1).

The abject is what "disturbs identity, system, order. What does not respect borders, positions, rules. The in-between, the ambiguous, the composite" (1982, p. 4), what separates the subject and threatens it (Brennan, 1993). It is a universal phenomenon, which can be found as soon as the symbolic dimension is formed, throughout civilizations, but which has specific forms, depending on the different cultures:

> A massive and sudden emergence of uncanniness, which, familiar as it might have been in an opaque and forgotten life, now harries me as radically separate, loathsome. Not me. Not that. But not nothing, either. A "something" that I do not recognize as thing. A weight of meaninglessness, about which there is nothing insignificant, and which crushes me. On the edge of non-existence and hallucination, of a reality that, if I acknowledge it, annihilates me. There, abject and abjection are my safeguards. The primers of my culture.
>
> (1982, p. 2)

This helps Kristeva describe how the abject manifested itself in certain social configurations. She indicates its role in the pagan rituals of impurity, its relevance in the different food taboos of monotheist religions, and the variations that the idea of original sin has impressed on the subject in Christianity. It is precisely in this last perspective that Kristeva locates the full subjective interiorization that refers, to use my terms, to the extimate nature of the law, decisive for Western culture:

> Christ is characterized and, as is well known, compels recognition in a most spectacular manner – superficial perhaps but striking. Those indications should not be construed as simply anecdotal or empirical, nor as drastic staging of a polemic with Judaism. What is happening is that a new arrangement of differences is being set up, an arrangement whose economy will regulate a wholly different system of meaning, hence a wholly different speaking subject.
>
> (1982, p. 113)

Christianity enabled a counterposition that operates in the subject itself. Through original sin, evil "displaced into the subject, will not cease tormenting him from within, no longer as a polluting or defiling substance, but as the ineradicable repulsion of his henceforth divided and contradictory being" (1982, p. 116). This condition, which essentially turns human beings into sinners – that feature that was confirmed with Adam's expulsion from Eden and which haunts all his descendants – will permit the greatest shows of love from the Creator. The possibility of soul salvation will reside there. So evil appears for the necessary unfolding of good, that is, as a kind of cornerstone of all possibility, such as the evil that unites men and women to the merciful Father. At this frontier, Kristeva encapsulates a large portion of the tribulations of modern subjectivity, which allows her to verify the eminently unique dimension of every social and political process, a question that she develops in *Intimate Revolt* [1997].

Such considerations on abjection take on even more importance if one considers Kristeva's developments from a linguistic perspective.[6] In works like "The Subject in Process" [1972] and *Revolution in Poetic Language* [1974], Kristeva distinguishes a first level of language linked with the primacy of the sign of a second level that she calls semiotic, which is related to the ineradicable heterogeneity harbored in each signifier.

Kristeva argues that the senses tend to overflow and modify the structural instances that order society due to their inherent multiplicity. Saussurean linguistics – unlike classical philology – noted this in stating that there is no closed system of signification; hence every language expresses an undecidable element. Poetic language is one expression where this is most evidently manifested. However, Kristeva argues that the semiotic level does not deny the symbolic function – even poetic language needs more than mere rhythm to exist – but rather there is no symbolic order without heterogeneity. Thus, Kristeva connects a post-structuralist approach with the most eminent developments of structuralism, since if it is a question of distinguishing what is unsustainable about the symbolic, nominal, paternal function, it would not be to the detriment of its enabling actions.

Consequently, this heterogeneity cannot be understood as a trace of the castrating action of the law, that is, an unwanted effect. What these considerations seem to confirm is the existence of a kind of pre-symbolic stage that replicates, in turn, these two levels of language. In other words, if the sign and the law are associated with the figure of the father, semiotics and heterogeneity are associated with the mother's. And the mother is tied to the body, a body that has not yet been bathed by language – what Kristeva (1998) alludes to with the term *chora*.[7] In *Desire in Language: A Semiotic Approach to Literature and Art*, she writes:

> The semiotic activity, which introduces wandering or fuzziness into a language, and *a fortiori* into poetic language is, from a synchronic point of view, a mark of the workings of drives (appropriation/rejection, orality/anality, love/hate, life/death) and, from a diachronic point of view, stems from the archaisms of the semiotic body. Before recognizing itself as identical in a mirror and, consequently, as signifying, this body is dependent vis-a-vis the mother. At the same time instinctual and maternal, semiotic processes prepare the future speaker for entrance into meaning and signification (the symbolic). But the symbolic (that is, language as nomination, sign, and syntax) constitutes itself only by breaking with this anteriority, which is

> retrieved as "signifier," "primary processes," displacement and condensation, metaphor and metonomy, rhetorical figures – but which always remains subordinate – subjacent to the principal function of naming-predicating.
>
> (1980, p. 136)

Having said this, the abject can only be thought of as an emergence of this primary, drive-oriented behavior, which is excluded with the aim of guaranteeing the organizational function of the signifier, that is, that first level of language that enables society. Joining this with the ideas in *Powers of Horror*, the abject can be understood as the irruption of the heterogeneous in signification, the symbolization of that which is, in fact, pre-symbolic, a Real anterior to the discursive – which brings us back to the knotting of Lacanian registers.

Certainly, Kristeva's approach has the merit of linking the ineradicable heterogeneity of the social with the lack and the attempts of the Symbolic to structure itself, but it also leaves open the chance to understand that its emergences are anterior, "natural", and that, therefore, they need to be assured or sustained, albeit marginally. Butler's critical stance in *Gender Trouble* [1990] expresses very well Kristeva's view, in that it "does not seriously challenge the structuralist assumption that the prohibitive paternal law is foundational to culture itself" (1999, p. 109). Thus, in Butler's view, Kristeva also fails to admit that the "subversion of paternally sanctioned culture cannot come from another version of culture, but only from within the repressed interior of culture itself, from the heterogeneity of drives that constitutes culture's concealed foundation" (1999, p. 110).

This criticism implies, in turn, another heuristic dimension: the impossibility of specifying the discursive production of the maternal body. For this reason, piggybacking Foucault, Butler notes that:

> Kristeva posits a maternal body prior to discourse that exerts its own causal force in the structure of drives, Foucault would doubtless argue that the discursive production of the maternal body as prediscursive is a tactic in the self-amplification and concealment of those specific power relations by which the trope of the maternal body is produced. In these terms, the maternal body would no longer be understood as the hidden ground of all signification, the tacit cause of all culture.
>
> (1999, p. 117)

This appraisal is relevant because it alludes to the background issue that shows the abject. Butler wonders whether those drives Kristeva speaks of, revealed only in language or in pre-established cultural forms, can actually come from a pre-symbolic dimension. Butler concludes that "[t]he multiple drives that characterize the semiotic constitute a prediscursive libidinal economy which occasionally makes itself known in language, but which maintains an ontological status prior to language itself" (1999, p. 102). In Butler's view, it is repression that creates the object that will be rejected as long as there is no instance that is not already informed by the norm or by the Symbolic. For this reason, Butler differs from Kristeva when she attempts to think of emancipation without a natural past to which one needs to return, with its "original pleasures", but rather to enable "an open future of cultural possibilities" (1999, p. 119).

Butler continues to explore this perspective in *Bodies That Matter* [1993]. There she denounces the naturalization of the norm, understanding the dangers of enshrining a sexual binarism as a natural definer of identities, which in turn implies the delimitation of degraded or excluded conditions within the terms of sociality. She notes how certain sexual expressions begin to be depicted as threats to the integrity of socially legitimate forms. In this context, the abject proves to be connected to the excluded of the Symbolic, but with no relation whatsoever to a stage preceding the Symbolic:

> The abject designates here precisely those "unlivable" and "uninhabitable" zones of social life which are nevertheless densely populated by those who do not enjoy the status of the subject, but whose living under the sign of the "unlivable" is required to circumscribe the domain of the subject. This zone of uninhabitability will constitute the defining limit of the subject's domain; it will constitute that site of dreaded identification against which – and by virtue of which – the domain of the subject will circumscribe its own claim to autonomy and to life. In this sense, then, the subject is constituted through the force of exclusion and abjection, one which produces a constitutive outside to the subject, an abjected outside, which is, after all, "inside" the subject as its own founding repudiation.
>
> (1993, p. xiii)[8]

The concept of abjection in Butler underlines the need to inquire into the reasoning of certain expressions that are not recognized in the symbolic order. This is, in fact, the subject that orients Butler's discussion with Lacan and Hegel's interpretations of the tragic character of Antigone.

Butler (2000) finds that both interpretations of the Greek heroine have a normalizing tone: In Lacan's case, given the primacy of the Oedipus complex; in Hegel's case, due to a state logic that is also patriarchal.[9] But what is interesting is that Butler's thematizations bring us back to the core of our inquiry into how to conceive the Real in politics. Indeed, in *Bodies That Matter*, Butler especially criticizes Laclau and Žižek's Lacanian stance on this concept, a question that is also found in the book on reciprocal interchanges titled *Contingency, Hegemony, Universality: Contemporary Dialogues on the Left* [2000]. In this book, Butler argues that to assume the Real as the impossible – as Laclau and Žižek do – is to nominate it directly, and in doing so, the Real not only appears as a limit of the Symbolic but also appears as a part of it, or better, as something integrated to it. Thus, she not only shows a distance from her interlocutors but also considers that this is the proper way the Real is to be understood in subjectivization processes.[10]

However, as Laclau comments, this assertion about the Real denotes an excessive trust in the capacity of the Symbolic. It even enables the possibility of thinking of a full representation or an identity between signifier and signified, something that, as Kristeva argues, is impossible.[11] To put it clearly: If one follows Butler in her view on the Real, that is, if one agrees with her statement that the Real is a part of the Symbolic in terms of a quasi-transcendental, what agency would the subject have to exceed the norm? How would a given field of representation be updated? In what way would a change in the social order occur? My aim with these questions is to show that Butler forgets that the Real is an impasse that is inherent to every formalization; hence, in her writings, the abject is either a contingent flaw of order or else an effect of order. But, in both cases, its existence seems avoidable as long as that portion of the norm that does not work is repaired, even when we know that the norm will never work perfectly. Quite plainly, it is as though in her criticism of the articulating effect of the Symbolic, Butler harbored a private and secret hope about the possibilities of order.[12]

As I said, I can only agree with Butler in her critique of Kristeva regarding the ever-symbolized dimension of the maternal, but I do not think it prudent to agree with her when she says the heterogeneous is a mere expression of the law, since this conspires to show the non-sense of any definition. It is true that her analyses make it possible to distinguish and denounce the naturalizations of exclusions – even the "biologization" of identity – but they also offer the chance to strengthen the same exclusions from an attempt to recompose the Symbolic. In recovering the agency and the ineradicable nature of the heterogeneous, Butler emphasizes that the heterogeneous can cease to be once it is acknowledged by order or in establishing a real democratic order that assumes an unlimited heterogeneity as a fundamental premise. To some extent, in reducing the Real to a moment of the Symbolic, the Real becomes liable to being returned to its true place, that is, to a place that makes its emergence impossible. Nonetheless, the problem is one of greater scope. It is necessary to understand that the impossibility is not of the Real but of the Symbolic. Hence, it is necessary to doubt the "male" and the "female", the "man" and the "woman", the "paternal" and the "maternal", and every other category or ordering pair, since its function and its actions enclose a non-sense but do not lead to a gross voluntarism.[13] Nor is it possible to isolate the Real from the Symbolic; only to seek the Real in the Symbolic, the Real from inside and outside, and to think of the specific manner in which the lack operates from the knot.

It is precisely this matter that does not seem to have been adequately considered, not only by Butler and Kristeva but also by several thinkers – all of them of utmost importance – of varied orientations, such as Gilles Deleuze and Félix Guattari (1983) in postulating the "Desiring-machine", Cornelius Castoriadis (1987) in thinking the "psychic monad", and even Lacanian thinkers such as Stavrakakis (2000, 2007), who has done enlightening work on the bond between psychoanalysis and politics.[14] What I mean by this is that it is most important to note the ontological assumptions of theoretical-political discourses to understand their corresponding perspectives. Indeed, some speak of emancipation as the purest resistance to power without conceiving the symbolic aspect that any effective policy entails – as we will see, Rancière's case is paradigmatic in this sense, but in a different sense, this is also true of Antonio Negri and Michael Hardt's case (2004). Thus, they are not capable of explaining how to articulate the heterogeneity of the identity points they invoke; they only postulate politics of scarce appeal or of impossible relevance to constitute an order with their own frontiers and exclusions.[15]

In the following chapter, I will explore Benjamin's work, suggesting another possible perspective for conceiving the Real or for finding the Real in political theory. I will attempt to show that his thinking on violence entails a pure Real that denies the eminently political dimension of existence. This will be crucial to understanding that abjection refers less to an act of exclusion than to a constitutive lack of the Symbolic that every act of exclusion seeks to block.

Notes

1 Alenka Zupančič also wrote an important work on this Freudian notion, although her work looks at the notion's connection with comedy: "We can now resume things by saying that what both comedy and the uncanny have in common has to do with – nothing" (2008, p. 50).

2 Fisher (2017) distinguishes the "weird" from the "eerie" when he says that the Freudian *Unheimliche* cannot capture aesthetic experiences marked by the sensation of an error coming from the outside. In associating the abject with the "extimate", my perspective argues with symbolic barriers precisely like those that Fisher aims to establish. In order to think in theoretical-political terms, I follow Kristeva here when she says that "[s]trangely enough, there is no mention of foreigners in the *Unheimliche*" (1991, p. 191). We may also recall that Dolar (1991) argues that Lacan invents the term extimacy as a way to translate the arguably ontological problem that Freud finds in the uncanny: "The English translation, 'the uncanny', largely retains the essential ambiguity of the German term, but French doesn't possess an equivalent, *l'inquiltante étrangeté* being the standard translation. So Lacan had to invent one: *extimité*" (Dolar, 1991, p. 6).

3 I put forward my position while referring again to the fundamental difference between Freud's and Lacan's views. For the former, the unconscious needs to be revealed; it means making the unconscious conscious; it means establishing an archeological perspective. For the latter, in contrast, the unconscious refers to extimacy and is therefore external to the subject in that the discourse of the Other exceeds it and precedes it. It is the scenario from which its life cannot escape. So in Lacan's view, but not Freud's, the word cannot find it, or the truth, it can only circumscribe it: "[F]or psychoanalysis, the unconscious is the indicator of a problem, of a conflict, of an

antagonism, and not simply and directly its (hidden) truth" (Zupančič, 2008, p. 16).

4 In Kafka's *The Metamorphosis* [1915], the main character Gregor Samsa awakes to find he has turned into a horrible insect. At no point does the reader find out the reason for this decisive process that modifies the nature of the character. Although he is still the same as ever, although he feels the same, Samsa notices he no longer is; he is no longer as he was. His family gradually begins to reject him, to exclude him from the symbolic field since his existence is unbearable to them, and they also begin to fear him. In fact, when he dies, they manage to restructure their lives without him, erasing the traces of his existence, and the sister and the parents feel liberated. How can we consider the abject aspects in this text? I would say that the abject does not lie in Samsa and his metamorphosis. Unlike what could be said with Freud, I do not believe that his transformation occurs because of the realization of a trauma, because of the emergence of something that was suppressed, his drives, or some other primary component that finds its destiny. The abject resides, in fact, in the position of the family, in their response to something that appears as monstrous or degraded, impossible to assimilate but constitutive of it (I owe this pertinent reflection to a thought-provoking comment by Alberto Fragio).

5 In his diary *De l'abjection* [1939], the anguished French writer Marcel Jouhandeau expressed how his homosexuality was connected to a deep Catholic religiousness. Eribon (2019) says that Jouhandeau follows mysticism as legitimation of the loss in sin; thus, it is necessary to become abject, to be worthy of God. Hence, abjection is sustained, as Bataille argues.

6 See Moi (1991).

7 The author takes the term from Plato's *Timaeus*. She understands it as an unnamable, unlikely receptacle, anterior to nomination, the One and the father, connoted as maternal. Derrida (1981) explored this notion in detail from another perspective.

8 Butler also addresses the abject in other titles, such as *Frames of War: When is Life Grievable?* [2009]– although without substantial additions or semantic variations.

9 I will revisit the figure of Antigone in my closing remarks.

10 In *Bodies That Matter*, Butler clearly says this: "To claim that the real resists symbolization is still to symbolize the real as a kind of resistance. The former claim (the real resists symbolization) can only be true if the latter claim ('the real resists symbolization' is a symbolization) is true, but if the second claim is true, the first is necessarily false. To presume the real in the mode of resistance is still to predicate it in some way and to grant the real its reality apart from any avowed linguistic capacity to do precisely that" (1993, p. 201).

11 As Laclau writes in *Contingency, Hegemony, Universality: Contemporary Dialogues on the Left*: "Butler perhaps is not advocating total representability – although it is difficult to see how the sublation of any 'non-representable' within the field of representation could lead to any different reading. Perhaps what she intends to point to is not a contradiction *sensu stricto* but a paradox – in that case she would be referring to an aporia

of thought, and we would be back to the terms of Russell's dilemma. The question there would be: what can we do when we are confronted with a discursive space organized around logically unanswerable aporias?" (2000, p. 67).

12 Ahmed (2000, 2004), who follows Butler on numerous matters, also gives too much sufficiency to the Symbolic. Indeed, it is precisely because of this that her perspective cannot access a notion of affectivity that might reveal how symbolic castration accounts for the impossibility of naming the event that occurs and reverberates in the body, and which differentiates it from the omnipotent trend of the discourse of the Other. I believe that, with its differences, this is something that follows other works that are part of the so-called *Affective Turn.*

13 I echo here Joan Copjec's pioneering criticism (1994) of a certain voluntarist assumption in Butler present in her early work. On this topic, I recommend consulting Sabsay (2016).

14 "In Lacan, this lack is, first of all, a lack of *jouissance*, the lack of a pre-symbolic, real enjoyment which is always posited as something lost, as a lost fullness, the part of ourselves that is sacrificed/castrated when we enter the symbolic system of language and social relations" (Stavrakakis, 2000, p. 41).

15 I would argue that, within the post-foundational universe, Laclau is one of the few thinkers – or even the only one – who escapes this criticism and who, rather, undertakes its challenge.

2 A Pure Real

Behind my argument about the unknotted nature of violence in Benjamin's interpretation – violence that appears as the Real with no symbolic inscription whatsoever – there is an underlying conceptual approach to understanding the ontology of politics. A reading of "Toward the Critique of Violence" reveals the importance of certain elements that refer to the status of abjection in the knotting of the three Lacanian registers. I suspect that with Benjamin's criticism of the relation between violence and the law, he ultimately disqualifies the question of the discourse of the political on the forms that any symbolic order takes, since ultimately his perspective leads to the denial of the Symbolic as such. This is a theoretical operation that differs from the one made by other thinkers mentioned earlier. For instance, as noted in the introduction, Butler reduces the Real to the ring of the Symbolic. As we shall see later, Agamben produces an imaginary expansion that subsumes the specificity of each of the strings with their knots, with their external and internal sections, that is, with their extimacy. This is not the case of Benjamin, who to some extent unties the Real from the Symbolic and the Imaginary and gives absolute autonomy to the Real, negating the knot itself.

Recall that from the outset of Benjamin's essay, he looks for an avenue of inquiry on violence that does not include the path of ethics. As he says, violence often appears in relation to justice and the law. This relationship is influenced by the question about the just or unjust nature of the ends and of the means used: Can a fair end make use of violence? Is violence an ethical means? If not, does its use block the characteristic of the perspective it seeks to contribute to? Benjamin argues that one must elude these questions when attempting to make a critique with disruptive capacity. Ultimately, violence is a means and not an end; hence, nothing can be definitively concluded in this field; it is necessary to suspend the question about justice and observe the violence in the law.[1]

Thus, Benjamin contrasts the tradition of natural law with that of positive law. He points out that according to the considerations of the former, violence is a natural matter, and hence it does not pose a problem provided the ends it serves are just. For the latter, on the other hand, violence appears as a historical

DOI: 10.4324/9781003457022-4

fact, whose complications are manifested when its use lacks legitimacy, that is, when violence is not endorsed within the margins of the legal system. Consequently, "if positive law is blind to the absoluteness of ends, natural law is equally so to the contingency of means" (2004, p. 237):

> Notwithstanding this antithesis, however, both schools meet in their common basic dogma: just ends can be attained by justified means, justified means used for just ends. Natural law attempts, by the justness of the ends, to "justify" the means, positive law to "guarantee" the justness of the ends through the justification of the means. This antinomy would prove insoluble if the common dogmatic assumption were false, if justified means on the one hand and just ends on the other were in irreconcilable conflict. No insight into this problem could be gained, however, until the circular argument had been broken, and mutually independent criteria both of just ends and of justified means were established.
>
> (2004, p. 237)

However, for Benjamin, there is a fundamental difference: While natural law provides a bottomless casuistry – hence, a critical inquiry into violence cannot be included in its domains – positive law allows us to address specific forms of violence. Benjamin argues that it is precisely on this path that the possibility of taking a stance on the very Weberian problem of the monopolization of physical coercion emerges. Indeed, he states that this prerogative does not seem to belong to the State. As we see later, Benjamin stresses that violence exceeds the logic of the law. Nonetheless, he is not at all concerned with discussing the background of this matter but rather emphasizing – and with it breaking – the recursion between law and violence.

It is well known that law uses violence to sustain itself, but it always leaves a possibility for a violent expression to occur that modifies its configuration or introduces a very different one in its place. Benjamin argues that this is the reason why the law cares less about the actions of criminals than about the legitimacy their actions may have. It is no coincidence that Benjamin highlights the danger of a criminal enjoying the people's affections. But this is not the greatest threat the law faces; its greatest danger stems from the prerogative to strike.

This situation shows that the workers who exercise it and the State that guarantees it are the only ones that can legitimately make use of violence. But it is clear that the workers are at a disadvantage: Their right to violence can always be revoked, even more so at the possibility of a strike becoming a "revolutionary general strike" (2004, p. 239). Hence, revolutionary attempts such as the Spartacist uprising cannot elude this legal recursion; on the contrary, they tend to strengthen it. Thus, violence comes boxed in a duality, or better still, it works as a kind of pendulum that swings between the law's capacity to instate or depose. Benjamin argues that evidence of this first form that violence can take comes from the right to war, while evidence of the second form comes from its most eminent continuation, militarism. In this context, he notes that both characteristics coexist in the police. The edicts that this institution formulates daily are part of the constant search to preserve the prevailing legal framework. However, Benjamin notes an interesting question:

> Unlike law, which acknowledges in the "decision" determined by place and time a metaphysical category that gives it a claim to critical evaluation, a consideration of the police institution encounters nothing essential at all. Its power is formless, like its nowhere-tangible, all-pervasive, ghostly presence in the life of civilized states. And though the police may, in particulars, appear the same everywhere, it cannot finally be denied that in absolute monarchy, where they represent the power of a ruler in which legislative and executive supremacy are united, their spirit is less devastating than in democracies, where their existence, elevated by no such relation, bears witness to the greatest conceivable degeneration of violence.
>
> (2004, p. 243)

On this point, Benjamin explores whether there is a way out of the predicament that implies that all violence as a means will be either law-making or law-preserving. He ponders:

> Is any nonviolent resolution of conflict possible? Without doubt. The relationships among private persons are full of examples of this. Nonviolent agreement is possible wherever a civilized outlook allows the use of unalloyed means of agreement. Legal and illegal means of every kind that are all the same violent may be confronted with nonviolent ones as unalloyed means. Courtesy, sympathy, peaceableness, trust, and whatever else might here be mentioned are their subjective preconditions. Their objective manifestation, however, is determined by the law (whose enormous scope cannot be discussed here) that says unalloyed means are never those of direct solutions but always those of indirect solutions.
>
> (2004, p. 244)

The law, with its violence, has infiltrated the mutual understanding between people, that is, in the very sphere of language, placing deception under punishment. But "it turns to fraud, therefore, not out of moral considerations but for fear of the violence that it might unleash in the defrauded party" (2004, p. 245).

After this statement, Benjamin returns to the matter of the strike, using the distinction that Georges Sorel established in his work *Reflections on Violence* [1908]: The political strike seeks to obtain substantial concessions and begin talks, while the proletarian general strike begins a process that seeks revolution. For this reason, Sorel was displeased with the mediations that could occur between will and the revolutionary event. Benjamin is aware of this. Sorel saw it as a spontaneous effect catalyzed by the myth, that is, by an image that could infuse moods in the workers so that they abandoned their work posts and set about the revolution. In fact, Sorel argues:

> A myth cannot be refuted since it is, at bottom, identical to the convictions of a group, being the expression of these convictions in the language of movement; and it is, in consequence, unanalysable into parts which could be placed on the plane of historical descriptions.
>
> (1999, p. 29)

Such considerations had a great influence in the first decades of the twentieth century. Authors of very diverse theoretical and political streams have used or discussed the ideas of this revolutionary syndicalist thinker. Gramsci, one of his keenest readers, dedicated numerous passages to him in *Prison Notebooks* [1919–1935]. In this text, the founder of the Italian Communist Party described Sorel as "anti-politicist".

In his perspective, Sorel merely rejected the need to coordinate the different social spheres and, in doing so, renounced the fundamental task of politics: the course of the "historic bloc", that is, hegemony. Following Lenin, Gramsci considered that the party of the masses should dispute control of a space of representation, patiently organizing insurrection. Hence, in his view, there was no room whatsoever for spontaneity. The force of the myth had to operate within a considered analysis of social conditions, a historical and objective analysis. But, in the work that concerns us here, Benjamin simply takes Sorel's conceptualization, adding that the proletarian general strike is the only possible way to end violence, the only instance that would turn violence into a "pure means", a "nonviolent" tool (2004, p. 246).

At this point in Benjamin's text, a number of questions have to be considered: How can we think of violence that is not tied to an end, that is, as "pure means"? How can we not think that the revolutionary general strike positions itself before the law, albeit only to achieve its aim of liquidating it? Why does Benjamin say, as we have seen, that actions made in the course of such a strike are not violent? The revolutionary general strike is not violent, Benjamin argues, because it seeks the end of the law. So violent acts that may occur in a strike appear as attempts to break the means-ends circularity. Thus, Benjamin believes he opens a new panorama. He says it is possible to trace marks that bear witness to a similar expression. In fact, the mythic violence described in Greek tragedies appears outside of the law.

In the verses of this artistic formulation of Antiquity, the judgment of the gods goes against the law established by men. On this point, Benjamin is compelled to swiftly clarify the nature of this violence. We could well suggest that this clarification is symptomatic of the complexity of violence as a study problem and even of the specificity of this problem in the German world. The fact that the term *gewalt*[2] encloses multiple and very dense meanings is a symptom of this. However, Benjamin clearly states that the violence of the gods observed in Greek tragedies refers to domination and to the scope of their authority; hence, it is a violence that competes in the same space as the law. Consequently, it does not break the connection denounced at the beginning of the essay. Benjamin poses the question about an immediate, pure violence that could end mythic violence. In decisive contrast, "divine violence" now appears:

> Just as in all spheres God opposes myth, mythic violence is confronted by the divine. And the latter constitutes its antithesis in all respects. If mythic violence is lawmaking, divine violence is law-destroying; if the former sets boundaries, the latter boundlessly destroys them; if mythic violence brings at once guilt and retribution, divine power only expiates; if the former threatens, the latter strikes; if the former is bloody, the latter is lethal without spilling blood.
>
> (2004, p. 249)

Benjamin says that "mythic violence is power over mere life for its own sake; divine violence is pure power over all life for the sake of the living. The first demands sacrifice; the second accepts it" (2004, p. 259). Thus:

> The educative power, which in its perfected form stands outside the law, is one of its manifestations. These are defined, therefore, not by miracles directly performed by God but by the expiating moment in them that strikes without bloodshed, and, finally, by the absence of all lawmaking. To this extent it is justifiable to call this violence, too, annihilating; but it is so only relatively, with regard to goods, right, life, and suchlike, never absolutely, with regard to the soul of the living. The premise of such an extension of pure or divine power is sure to provoke, particularly today, the most violent reactions, and it to be countered by the argument that, if taken to its logical conclusion, it confers on men even lethal power against one another. This, however, cannot be conceded.
>
> (2004, p. 250)

Critic Hamacher (1991) comments that divine violence is *afformative*, not performative; that is to say, it does not imply any realization or representation. It is "the event of forming, itself formless, to which all forms and all performative acts remain exposed" (1991, p. 1139). Hence his consideration that Benjamin succeeds in bringing about a "reversal of the perspective of classic political theory" (1991, p. 1154), a tradition greatly concerned with the production of regimes and government systems that seek social harmony of the whole community. Hamacher argues that the proletarian general strike is not directed toward any object or objective, nor is it "directed toward *nothing*"; hence, it "can be described as being without intention" (1991, p. 1147). That is, it is "a nonaction", "as an unconditional refusal to act it is tantamount to a 'severing of relations'" (1991, p. 1149).

Hamacher does not find a theological remainder in Benjamin's ideas, much less a heterodox, Messianic approach; nothing is expected of the revolutionary general strike; it is pure suspension. However, Hamacher admits that the strike implies a certain form of political affiliation, even if it cannot be defined, since it refers to politics as such:

> Not as a particular form of politics, but as a manifestation of the political as such, and of the only contemporary political force recognized by Benjamin, the proletariat, not as the application of one political means among others, but as an event of the mediacy of the political itself, the strike would suspend any politics oriented toward violently posited ends, and would thus itself be the sheer medium of the political: the only politics which does not serve as an instrument. With the proletarian strike, with the deposing of the rule of positive law, the imparting structure of language, the social itself would historically break through and open up another history.
>
> (1991, p. 1150)[3]

Hamacher sees a certain anarchist position in Benjamin, at least in this 1920s text. I would argue that aside from observing some modulations and indications of this, what is interesting is to understand Benjamin's approach based on the problem of abjection. In this context, the first thing to note – following Hamacher – is that it is very significant that Benjamin's work on violence appears as a "political" text; it is very interesting because it is Benjamin who, in my view, renounces thinking the mediations inherent to politics. I would say that Hamacher finds the way for the "political" in Benjamin to dispense with its constitutive dimensions. It is as though Benjamin were speaking about a kind of "ontological politics", a fundamental ontology, without symbolic or historical derivations. In my view, Hamacher's problem is that he ultimately shifts the "political" in Benjamin to the register of history without assuming the historical abjections. Only this way can the denunciation of the law be understood as the possibility of a rupture that is still political but which lacks entirely the particularistic features of politics. Thus, it is feasible to think that Hamacher's reading associates Benjamin with a certain nihilism, even despite himself. To put it plainly, violence as a pure means leads to an instance about which nothing can be said or predicated. Benjamin speaks to us about a specific violence, whose specificity or particularity consists, however, of not being a particular expression, that is, equal to any other. But where does the divine of this violence lead?

This suspicion provides the grounds for those perspectives that claim the presence of a messianic dimension in Benjamin's arguments – let us consider Agamben (1999a) as one example. Such readings are often reinforced with Benjamin's posthumous text, "Theses on the Philosophy of History", written between 1939 and 1940. Without seeking to explore this dense debate, my intention is only to point out that in 1921, the messianic is necessarily questioned when it is aligned with Benjamin's anti-sovereign stance. However, what truly interests me in this whole matter is that divine violence excludes meaning. It is merely the violence of an untied pure Real, which leads politics to its dissolution, its extinction, since it suspends every symbolic mediation, every imaginary support, it blocks the lack, it eliminates it from the outside. And here, there is a similarity with any paradigm that positions in a future of action the negation of the political. So in simple terms, *if Hamacher postulates that Benjamin, in referring to violence from the register of afformativeness, refers to politics as such, I maintain, from a Lacanian non-ontology, that his entire conception in that regard leads to a denial of politics as such.*

For this reason, it is relevant to note that Benjamin, arguing against the justification of murder in the Ten Commandments, said that "neither the divine judgment, nor the grounds for this judgment, can be known in advance" (2004, p. 250). He also noted:

> Less possible and also less urgent for humankind, however, is to decide when unalloyed violence has been realized in particular cases. For only mythic violence, not divine, will be recognizable as such with certainty, unless it be in incomparable effects, because the expiatory power of violence is invisible to men. Once again all the eternal forms are open to pure divine violence, which myth bastardized with law.
>
> (2004, p. 252)

This, which can be deemed another influence of Sorel's vitalism and Benjamin's Jewish roots, takes on considerable nuance from the question of abjection. It could be speculated that the difficulty in recognizing divine violence, which leaves subjects in the radical contingency of ignorance – which in turn stresses the critique of the Greek inheritance, which, together with Christianity, built the idea that fate is inexorable, as Benjamin writes[4] – leads to a retreat on what the proletarian general strike actually means. Consequently, it would appear that the view of violence as a pure means leads to the suspension of the symbolic order as such, and hence, it shuts down the question of abjection.

This may be the reason why it is difficult to recognize when divine violence is manifested; perhaps because of this, Benjamin introduces it as an expression that is not theological and does not draw on the law, as a violence that disqualifies the structure of discursiveness and is always inscribed in it. Thus, the Real of violence is ultimately inherent to an order that is not an order that is not perforated.[5]

In *Force of Law* [1994], Jacques Derrida addressed this same difficulty of distinguishing mythic violence from divine violence following Benjamin's curious statement on the impossibility of fully grasping what each of them consists of. Provocatively, Derrida (1992) linked this feature of violence with its destructive nature. According to Derrida, Benjamin's perspective could well lead to something similar to the Final Solution advocated by Nazism.

In contrast, Butler (2020) finds therein the principle of non-violence, a most remarkable discovery since it greatly eludes the terms introduced by Benjamin himself. In turn, Agamben (2005) used this same difficulty of recognition to argue that Benjamin refers to a time in which there is no longer an exception or any rule whatsoever. Hence, Benjamin may have used a messianic violence to break with the death machinery inherent to the paradigm of sovereignty. In my case, I have a very different reading of Benjamin's text: The violence that appears there as pure means is no more than an untied Real that can neither speak about the political and its uniqueness nor explain the gap of abjection. Thus, despite Derrida's claim, I do not believe that Benjamin's words can be linked to Nazi extermination, as in lacking any symbolic inscription; his writing ultimately negates every historical sedimentation of politics.

This distance allows us to assert that there is no social order without the knotting between the Real, the Symbolic, and the Imaginary. There is no order whatsoever, no symbolic stabilization, without an extimate Real that constitutes it and threatens it; without that impossible place of representation of the lack of object that Lacan talked about. The figures I will refer to later will bear witness to different modalities postulated by contemporary political discourses to deal with it. The first one, Sacrifice, which has such a connection with the religious and theological dimension, will be addressed based on the critical imputations on sovereignty included in the writings of Girard and Agamben.

Notes

1 It is significant that the precaution on ethics is echoed in this text by Benjamin as well as in Weber's lecture (2004), which took place at about the same time, dealing with politics as vocation. In both, the ethical question is stressed but then later suspended, a highly relevant matter when it comes to understanding their corresponding analyses.
2 The term can be translated as "violence", "force", "power", and "authority".
3 It is interesting to note that in "On Language as Such and on the Language of Man" [1916] – a text that is often used to address some of the more complex points of "Toward the Critique of Violence" – Benjamin points out that the symbolic order of humans derives – with all its peculiarities – from divine order, appearing as a precarious translation of what God has created with his word. As we shall see, in "Toward the Critique of Violence", that need appears suspended, marked as futile due to the unspeakable.
4 This particular reading can be observed by taking as reference the mention of the myth of Niobe, present in the text that concerns us here, in the reflections on "Fate and Character" [1919] and on "Capitalism as Religion" [1921].
5 In *Violence: Six Sideways Reflections*, Žižek portrays Benjamin's divine violence as a violence without the guarantee of the big Other, and he mirrors Alain Badou's notion of "Event" (2005). It is interesting that, from a different register, Jesi (2000) portrays uprisings as a moment of truth in that everything that happens therein acquires that status due to the sheer weight of events.

Part Two

Sacrifice

3 The Crisis of Distinctions

René Girard addressed violence in a number of his works, such as *Violence and the Sacred* [1972] and *The Scapegoat* [1982], highlighting sacrifice as an institution that permitted its regulation. However, toward the end of his life, he made an interesting change in this regard. His book *Achever Clausewitz* [2007] – translated into English as *Battling to the End* – was no longer concerned with the contrast between archaic and modern societies; the important aspect had ceased to be the penetration of the sacred in the social and its connection with violence or the justification of why, in a secularized world, it was imperative to develop some sort of device to administer it. Now it was a question of avoiding the destruction of life as a result of the Atomic Age; that is, it was a question of negating any violent presence in the community, highlighting the satanic root of sacrifice, the danger of a total, collective sacrifice. However, in this 2007 text, and in spite of its marked religious tone, Girard was able to reinforce something already present in his preceding texts: the crucial and irrepressible dimension of violence.

In the past, as in the present, humanity only reproduced violent forms of social bond, sometimes seeking to deal with that same violence, sometimes unleashing it in unprecedented ways, in great wars, in mass slaughters of men and women. In both cases, violence is a problem that questions the political. I will attempt to understand here how Girard, in the aforementioned works, went from analyzing an apparent form of abjection and comparing it with another to rejecting any kind of abjection or, in Lacanian terms, rejecting the experience of the lack, denying that which endangers the consistency of the Borromean knot.

At first, Girard maintained the centrality of the sacred in the social, stating that political order should be articulated around this principle. But he then denied the validity of any political order, arguing that the social should become the sacred, or, indeed, that the sacred should be the same thing as the social. This transition in Girard solely interests me in considering how the figure of sacrifice alludes to a certain solidarity that the religious (or the theological) holds with the political in diverse contemporary authors of great importance in contemplating contemporary politics.

DOI: 10.4324/9781003457022-6

In his work about Clausewitz, Girard portrays a kind of absolutization of the Real, no longer from violence – that which in his preceding works showed the failure of the Symbolic without denying it – but because of the relevance of Christ. The Messiah turns out to be the very expression of truth and the absolute. Christ is the Real, which shall prevail in reality, the one who showed the world the path to extinction of every conflictive emergency of human life, of every germ of violence. To be more precise, he is *the* Real that annuls the Real of violence with its diabolical institutions – such as sacrifice – or lapsed institutions – such as sovereignty and the State. For this reason, this "second" or "last" Girard uses a Real that does not admit cracks in the Symbolic, does not explain the Symbolic, but rather demands its annulment. For that to occur, a type of religious discourse has to prevail that has already been revealed and that can annul the abjection of the sin, unlike what Kristeva says in her renowned essay. This is why Girard does not ultimately consider violence a manifestation of the divine, but its simplest denial; this is why he neither turns the Real into an unanchored Real, whose power is extra-human, nor represents it as a Real that must be realized with the religious conversion of humanity.

In his early inquiries into it in 1972, Girard indicates a certain paradox of sacrifice:

> Because the victim is sacred, it is criminal to kill him – but the victim is sacred only because he is to be killed. Here is a circular line of reasoning that at a somewhat later date would be dignified by the sonorous term ambivalence.
>
> (1989, p. 1)

Thus, he makes a kind of comparison between violence and the sacred. He argues that such elements are articulated at the origin of all social life. He sustains that scientific paradigms and dominant ideologies have sought to deny this founding nature, even underestimating it by relegating religion to the margins of the private sphere. Hence, Girard seeks to highlight the importance of an approach that positions the sacred at the center of the social, that is, at the center of an explanation on the social itself; a secret center, evidently, which hides a truth: Any foundational act entails violence and death.

In referring to the ancient institution of sacrifice and its vitality in the societies of old time, Girard takes a position on the true beginning of community life. In doing so, he begins to show what is implied in the unfolding of the political, as though its most primitive tasks were directed toward doing something with the violence that invariably circulates in each person. Sacrifice is, in fact, an institution destined for this task.

Thus, Girard uses an original philosophical anthropology that enables him to establish a critique of the typically modern way of dealing with violence. This is merely an excuse to express a whole distance with the very ideals of Modernity, perhaps reducible to a paradigm of equality or leveling between individuals.

In this regard, Girard says little about the actual history of the individual; his method makes it an abstraction, as if men and women had always been conceived the same way, throughout centuries and civilizations. Girard does not do as Hegel, who was so persistent in showing the deployment and the alibis of the ideas of freedom; instead, he resembles his old counter-revolutionary compatriots, who centuries ago warned of the indistinctness that trampled on medieval order, so closely ruled by theological justifications. With good reason, Joseph de Maistre (1993) is a true authority on sacrifice. In a treatise, he argued that sacrifice has always existed and will always exist in all societies. Nonetheless, Girard was less concerned with this regularity in history that Maistre saw than with carrying out an operation in anachronism that would serve him as an accurate point of attack against Modernity – a Modernity that, in his words, was determined to continue on an unstoppable path of leveling and, therefore, one of incapacity to maneuver against violence. In fact, this road would lead to an unstoppable spiral. From his perspective, there is no society without violence. Community life forms an unbreakable tie with this primary, destructive, and ambiguous element. In fact, as an institution, sacrifice implies rites and routines that show the frontier between the sacred and the profane.

To prepare the sacrificial victim with certain provisions shows the considered intention of the community to please the gods, stopping them from unleashing their fury on the land, the crops, and the settlers. Girard acknowledges that all this encloses a mystification: Sacrifice is a device that regulates violence, allowing a symbolic stabilization of what seems to escape law or order, of what disrupts or tears the community fabric. It is an act filled with violence that seeks to avoid the uncontrolled violence of the social. The ritualized murder of a victim, carefully selected and prepared for it, contains the rage circulating among individuals and prevents it from disintegrating the space they share. Sacrifice produces a point of condensation of violence, which invokes the internal threat that violence represents for the social:

> Where only shortly before a thousand individual conflicts had raged unchecked between a thousand enemy brothers, there now reappears a true community, united in its hatred for one alone of its number. All the rancors scattered at random among the divergent individuals, all the differing antagonisms, now converge on an isolated and unique figure.
>
> (1989, p. 79)

In archaic societies, there is a kind of "sacrificial substitution" (1989, p. 5), that is, a real shift that means that the device deployed does not lose effectiveness; on the contrary, it is precisely here that the heart of the operation lies:

> Sacrifice plays a very real role in these societies, and the problem of substitution concerns the entire community. The victim is not a substitute for some particularly endangered individual, nor is it offered up to some individual

> of particularly bloodthirsty temperament. Rather, it is a substitute for all the members of the community, offered up by the members themselves. The sacrifice serves to protect the entire community from *its own* violence; it prompts the entire community to choose victims outside itself. The elements of dissension scattered throughout the community are drawn to the person of the sacrificial victim and eliminated, at least temporarily, by its sacrifice.
>
> (1989, p. 8)

In order for the sacrifice to be useful, its violence must be forgotten or unknown, and, thus, the social origin must be lost. Only then, only after forgetting, will it be possible to evoke it: "Indeed, the formidable effectiveness of the process derives from its depriving men of knowledge: knowledge of the violence inherent in themselves with which they have never come to terms" (1989, p. 82). In fact, its very simple mechanics benefits it: A "surrogate victim" (1989, p. 79) is chosen – a male, female, or animal figure that is part of the community – and, after a series of specific rituals, it is killed, thus transforming it into an offering to the Gods:

> The sacrificial process requires a certain degree of misunderstanding. The celebrants do not and must not understand the true role of the sacrificial act. The theological basis of the sacrifice has a crucial role in fostering this misunderstanding. It is the god who supposedly demands the victims; he alone, in principle, who savors the smoke from the altars and requisitions the slaughtered flesh. It is to appease his anger that the killing goes on, that the victims multiply.
>
> (1989, p. 7)

But Girard reaffirms that sacrifice does not calm divine fury or bless the community for its obedience since its function is very different and has nothing to do with atonement. "Rather, society is seeking to deflect in a relatively indifferent victim, a 'sacrificeable' victim, the violence that would otherwise be vented on its own members, the people it most desires to protect" (1989, p. 4). Hence, violence is intertwined with the sacred but does not have its true inscription there, its authentic *raison d'être*. Sacrifice is a real institution that revolves around an illusory entity. This means the illusion is not entirely false because, through its use, an extimate dimension to the community is apparently constituted. That is to say, sacrifice creates a limit point for symbolic order. While violence is brought together and released at the same time, in the same form and toward a single target, the victim shows the artificiality; hence, it is not the abject; it is the imaginarization of abjection. However, with Girard, we can see that the sacrificial victim expresses a way of relating with the decidedly foreign, which runs through the question that abjection reveals, since there is an estrangement that is no such thing. An Other is forged that unifies that which threatens to disunite everything.

In archaic communities, as I said, the sacrificial justification is religious, but its effectiveness is eminently political, despite its legitimations and discourses of solidarity. In Girard's view, theology as a register that enables the comprehension of this process should not be abandoned, nor should it be meekly accepted. Girard argues that it is necessary to criticize it to recover the conflictive relations that are intertwined between the theological and the political. Consequently, he does not follow the path of Hubert and Mauss (1964). In simple terms, although he agrees with these authors on its social nature, Girard does not agree that sacrifice is a ritual mechanism that lifts fundamental prohibitions without suppressing them, establishing at the same time a logic of representation of shared intuitions, perceptions, and beliefs.[1] He argues that nor is it a device that should be considered successful; rather, in the past, it played a function in something ineradicable in human nature and which might bring the demise of community life.[2] Consequently, his 1972 text does not attempt to reclaim it as a tool for the twentieth century; he merely highlights the closeness archaic societies maintained with that background that gives life to any human group, unlike the "evolved" groups of Modernity.

Indeed, Girard states in Modernity a real "sacrificial crisis" (1989, p. 39) has emerged that threatens the stabilization of every form of life. Differences between individuals have already been entirely diluted, as though they were irrelevant or should be censored. Sovereignty, as an organizational paradigm of the political, only negates the religious root of the social and fails to recognize the exclusions that must necessarily occur for any order to be stable. In a world that prides itself on its crucial secularized nature, sacrifice has no place except in the archives of barbarity. But barbarity – true barbarity, Girard argues – prevails under other masks, perhaps under the masks that reason establishes from a false moral authority. Thus, the violence of the social can no longer be managed by an institution that ties together the religious and the profane, the individual and the collective. Violence becomes a phenomenon that relies only on the inhabitants of the community; that is, it is explained by an anomaly whose responsibility lies with each person. In other words, modern society no longer considers itself violent or sacred; less still does it assume the inherent elements that make it and threaten it from its bowels. It only wants, Girard argues, to present violence as a marginal, random, pathological manifestation that affects the lives of those private individuals who are one way or another involved, contingently or randomly, in conflictive events. In short, there is a privatization of violence, a privatization of its most pure ontological negation.

In this context, the modern legal system contains one fundamental error. Its actions always occur after a violent event; it only seeks to remedy the damage suffered by the victim. It is not anticipatory. The symbolic cost is paid by whoever is found guilty, according to the provisions of the legal codes. Hence, unlike the Italian Middle Ages with their never-ending wars between families, disturbing the whole city, the modern State started to concern itself with disputes by institutionalizing revenge, turning it into the essence of justice, though failing to prevent or direct violence. Consequently, responsibility no longer lies with the community; there is no longer transcendence that replicates events; there is no longer any social distinction, only pure homogenization, only ungovernable atoms. The ideal of equality has triumphed, and, in Girard's view, only its severe consequences can be verified:

> The sacrificial crisis, that is, the disappearance of the sacrificial rites, coincides with the disappearance of the difference between impure violence and purifying violence. When this difference has been effaced, purification is no longer possible and impure, contagious, reciprocal violence spreads throughout the community.
>
> The sacrificial distinction, the distinction between the pure and the impure, cannot be obliterated without obliterating all other differences as well. One and the same process of violent reciprocity engulfs the whole. The sacrificial crisis can be defined, therefore, as a crisis of distinctions – that is, a crisis affecting the cultural order. This cultural order is nothing more than a regulated system of distinctions in which the differences among individuals are used to establish their "identity" and their mutual relationships.
>
> (Girard, 1989, p. 49)

If we analyze in depth the figure of "surrogate victim" discussed by Girard in his first texts, we will see that it encloses several interesting features to understand the characterization that the author offers of the present or, at least, of the historical context that has unfolded since the second half of the twentieth century.

As he notes, it is a question of a member of the community who must be removed for their subsequent sacrifice. Their sacred condition encloses a paradox: Since the future victim is sacred, they cannot be murdered, but only when their murder is perpetrated by society do they become a transcendental figure of the community. In the next chapter, I will show how this ambivalence, which Girard emphasizes, is also stressed by Agamben, who notes the theological dimension of the political with the figure of the *homo sacer*. But, unlike Agamben, Girard sees in the victim a point of condensation of different pairs – sacred/profane, divine/mundane, public/private – and not an indistinction. Thus, it is not a question of a lack of symbolic or imaginary frontiers that turn the exception into the rule, as in Agamben; it is a matter of a complex place from which the lack of any specific political definition is observed. It could be said that Girard does not tolerate the absence of a criterion that operates without consideration. Nonetheless, there is no part of his thinking marked by a gesture of solidarity with a defense of the political decision; on the contrary, he denounces the consequences of the specific prevalent political form in Modernity. Or, more reservedly, he denounces modern political organization, since, as we have seen, it all leads to the multiplication *ad infinitum* of violent points that threaten social life. Thus, to be quite clear, what has failed in Modernity is none other than the fact of omitting or avoiding the very root that explains the origin of the community, an organization that denies it.

Even if one were to argue that Girard looks on the pre-modern world with nostalgia, it must be remembered that the first precedent of the sacrificial crisis he describes occurred many centuries before. In the tragic tales of Antiquity there appeared, according to his research, the elements that best explain the implications that are the tonic of Modernity. In fact, in a work such as *Oedipus Rex,* it is possible to see the indistinction that wholly marks the twentieth century.

In Girard's view, the great theme that Sophocles expressed is none other than the difficulty in distinguishing violence and, thus, the possibility of understanding its social responsibility. Consequently, who murdered Layo would not be so relevant, for instance, as all the characters in the plot – even the king killed by his son – reacted with rage, living with violence, unable to give it up. This is the symptom of the crisis of order as a whole. In such an extreme, degenerated environment, there is no way of understanding what it is that distinguishes individuals, what sets the good apart from the bad, the innocent from the guilty:

> As in Greek tragedy and primitive religion, it is not the differences but the loss of them that gives rise to violence and chaos, that inspires Ulysses' plaint. This loss forces men into a perpetual confrontation, one that strips them of all their distinctive characteristics – in short, of their "identities". Language itself is put in jeopardy. "Each thing meets/In mere oppugnancy": the adversaries are reduced to indefinite objects, "things" that wantonly collide with each other like loose cargo on the decks of a storm-tossed ship. The metaphor of the floodtide that transforms the earth's surface to a muddy mass is frequently employed by Shakespeare to designate the undifferentiated state of the world that is also portrayed in Genesis and that we have attributed to the sacrificial crisis.
>
> (1989, p. 51)

But Girard says that the Greeks, unlike modern people, had their *pharmakos*, that is, their "venom" and their "antidote", generally in the same person. Thus, Oedipus is the *pharmakos* of Thebes, though not because of the parricide or the incest he unwittingly committed, but because of his condition of "scapegoat" (Girard, 1986). The whole community considers him guilty for the plague that subjugates old and young, women and children with the fist of death. Thus, even if still a hero, a savior, Oedipus cannot be sacrificed; he is not, in fact, killed in a ritual, but rather it is he himself who chooses his path of atonement, being consumed in the duality of the *pharmakos.* As we know, he chooses self-mutilation and ostracism. He carries out a just sentence. From my analytical perspective, this variation that Girard finds suggests the need to readjust the margins of comprehension of the political, for the work of Sophocles may reveal an utterly instructive reflection on knowledge and power, only capable of being fully understood from the problem of the relation between secret and politics.[3]

Girard's interpretation of the figure of Oedipus is highly relevant as it mobilizes the disciplinary diatribes that mark *Violence and the Sacred.* Girard turns this tragic hero into a true catalyst who fails to explain the individual conscience as Freud intended or the prohibitive dimension of incest that Claude Lévi-Strauss stresses. Possessive of the uniqueness of his reading, Girard notes that it is not the myth of the neurotic nor the myth that structures community order that Oedipus shows; Oedipus is, above all, a figure, a key modality of the social, which, for that same reason, cannot be corroborated by history, aside from the popular myths and tales that circulated about him in Antiquity.

Hence, here the unavoidable question arises of the method deployed by Girard; a question, however, that is not for us to pursue to its ultimate consequences, although we must ground it properly: What is the heuristic value of a view that is inscribed in a particular type of philosophical anthropology that dispenses with the burden of past events and their interpretations? Bluntly speaking, this is not a fundamental question that may trouble Girard; indeed, he seems quite unconcerned with the capacity to contrast his hypothesis. However, it is necessary in order to understand the limits he establishes with other approaches and authors. To some extent, Girard merely approaches his much admired, and debated, Freud, especially Freud's statements about the primitive horde. It is no coincidence that he explicitly argues with the theories present in another Freudian text, *Totem and Taboo* [1913], arguing that the murder of the father is far from the beginning of morals, religion, and guilt, but rather it is sacrifice that truly enables the social.

This does not effectively explain what the origin of violence is. Girard is well aware of this. Probably for this reason, he writes an answer based on the mimetic dimension of desire.

To be clear, "Mimetic Desire" (1989, p. 143) explains the proliferation and contagion that leads to the proliferation of violence. Girard seems to come close here to Hegel's considerations on recognition while openly affirming his distance from him. He maintains that there is no dialectic possible between desire and violence. It is curious that the well-known depth of the Hegelian considerations does not prompt him to say much. Moreover, he does not delve into the teachings of Lacan to resume or settle his hypotheses – teachings that, informed by the work of Kojève (1980) on *The Phenomenology of Spirit*, thought desire as "desire of the Other". It would seem that Girard only wanted to confront Freud and point out that he was able to resume what Freud unwisely discarded. From Girard's perspective, the mimesis of desire resembles the process of identification that Freud pointed out, a process that is based on the Oedipus complex and which entails a true affective bond between parents and child. The great distance that Girard claims – in a clear reductionism of the Freudian work – lies in that nothing related to desire comes from the unconscious of the subject or from its singular psychic constitution. The question is, in truth, eminently social.

Girard introduces important variations on these matters in *Battling to the End*, a book of conversations with the French literary critic and playwright Benoît Chantre. There Girard returns to Clausewitz's work, maintaining that in the twentieth and early twenty-first centuries, it is no longer a question of regulating violence, less still doing so in the manner of archaic societies studied in his early works; rather, it is a matter of fully refuting sacrifice and, in doing so, violence itself.

In this context, Girard suggests that men and women should abandon the mimesis of desire and identify only with the one whom they should truly follow, namely, Christ. Only the religion that takes Jesus as the one chosen by the Creator can overcome the sacrificial crisis inherent to Modernity and block the emergence of any violent manifestation on Earth. In this regard, Girard claims that Christianity neither enables nor tolerates sacrifice, hence nor does it resemble Judaism and its failed sacrifice of Isaac – the sacrifice that God asks of Abraham but which he does not carry out in the end. For this reason, Girard maintains that if religion invents sacrifice, Christianity deprives it of it. Thus, the author goes back on his words, and what he may have considered an effective way to regulate violence at some point in his career appears now judged as satanized, contrary to the sacred and befitting the purest pagan barbarity.[4]

This return of religion that Girard openly suggests has a flip side – once again – of the evident failure of politics. In his view, the politics of sacrifice failed, as did the politics of sovereignty. In this context, it is not a question of restoring the church, but an intimate, almost mystic connection of each and every human with God. He considers that Clausewitz – whom I will refer to later when discussing the figure of war from Schmitt's considerations – was the first modern author to notice the monumental escalation of violence that would mark the following centuries and its possible reversion.

Girard understands Clausewitz in a very different way from other great contemporary interpreters, such as Basil Liddell Hart (2012), who saw Clausewitz as merely a fanatic, and Raymond Aron (1983), who saw him as a rationalist. In Girard's view, the author of *On War* was an astute thinker who showed the "escalation to extremes" (2010, p. 1) but who abandoned his accurate intuitions due to his decisive consideration of the political conduct of hostilities. This judgment coincides with what Girard had already formulated on the institutionalization of revenge and the sacrificial crisis: All signs suggest, in his view, that the destruction of humanity is a certain possibility, even more so in the nuclear era. For this reason, revisiting Schmitt, he believes that it is no longer about gestating a politics of the exceptional or about enabling a decision that makes law and life possible; violence has already surpassed every norm, every possibility of imposition.[5] The mimesis of desire must be exchanged by a mimesis with Christ who, with his death, sought to block the possibility of any conflict in the world:

> However, in a world where the founding murder has disappeared, we have no choice but to imitate Christ, imitate him to the letter, do everything he says to do. The Passion reveals both mimetism and the only way to remedy it.
>
> (2010, p. 101)

Thus, we are in the presence of a realization of an unbarred big Other, of an order that fails to recognize the Real, of a primacy of the Imaginary register:

> By accepting crucifixion, Christ brought to light what had been "hidden since the foundation of the world," in other words, the foundation itself, the unanimous murder that appeared in broad daylight for the first time on the cross. In order to function, archaic religions need to hide their founding murder, which was being repeated continually in ritual sacrifices, thereby protecting human societies from their own violence. By revealing the founding murder, Christianity destroyed the ignorance and superstition that are indispensable.
>
> Freed of sacrificial constraints, the human mind invented science, technology and all the best and worst of culture. Our civilization is the most creative and powerful ever known, but also the most fragile and threatened because it no longer has the safety rails of archaic religion. Without sacrifice in the broad sense, it could destroy itself if it does not take care, which clearly it is not doing.
>
> (2010, p. XIII)

Girard trusts that, sooner or later, men and women will renounce violence without sacrifice, or else they will destroy the planet: "Humanity will be either in a state of grace or in mortal sin" (2010, p. 21). In fact, he asserts that the time of the Apocalypse has already started – the true and likely ultimate chance for humanity to make a change in its way of living.[6]

The sacred, then, can reappear decidedly, marking the true order of the human. In 2007 – when this last Girard work was published – there was no longer any impossibility of that, simply because the Real was no longer defined as violence but as religion, as the true religion. This needed to reappear as the cornerstone, as the justification for a society that differed from the modern one and the sacrificial one of old. Thus, the very plane of abjection, of the Real in its extimate relation with the Symbolic, would disappear, would be erased from the globe.[7]

In Agamben's discourse, in turn, the figure of sacrifice tied to the sacred is not portrayed as the opposition to sovereignty, as its other, but as its actual justification. From his perspective, it is not a question of thinking about the relation that is established with the truth of origin but of showing the indetermination that it generates, that is, a very specific form of politics that gives rise to a death machine.

Notes

1 "Let us try to uncover the societal conflicts that the sacrificial act and its theological interpretations at once dissimulate and appease. We must break with the formalistic tradition of Hubert and Mauss" (Girard, 1989, p. 7).
2 Could it be that Girard is thinking, via certain digressions, about the old Hobbesian problem of civil war or the state of nature that spurred the debate on sovereignty, even in Schmittian terms?
3 I am currently working on a book about secrecy from an ontological-political reading of *Oedipus Rex* and centering on the problem of order and authority.
4 Curiously, from the figure of sacrifice, it is possible to assert something contrary to Girard's ideas, since Christ effectively sacrificed himself for humanity. This has sustained the theological discourse. He did it to fulfill his divine mission, which closely ties humanity with God, after the disobedience of Adam and Eve. As is known, in the New Testament, God never appears before Jesus or speaks to him to directly request such a mission. There is a dimension of interpretation that only Christ as mediator carries out and which possesses an eminently political aspect: The absolute is lost; it is only revealed in the word, and this word originates interpretation. In Abraham, on the other hand, God explicitly requests the sacrifice of his son and then, on seeing his obedience, tells him not to do it through the intervention of an angel, who stops his arm right before it is stained with the murder of his offspring. These two modalities of sacrifice express, then, very different aspects. If Oedipus is also added, we see an even more complex and heterodox panorama. Oedipus is not the son who must be sacrificed – but will not be – at the request of a demanding God, who claims obedience in the foundation of his chosen people; nor is he the son who sacrifices himself at the request of the father for the benefit of a generic other such as one made up of men and women, including those to come; Oedipus sacrifices himself after the murder of his father; he may even sacrifice himself for having committed a sacrifice that is not. Nonetheless, Oedipus's sacrifice does not lead to his own death, only his mutilation. I consider that Derrida (1996) does not adequately contemplate these differences when thinking about the relation between ethics and the secret running through the history of Abraham. The unfathomable decision is only possible if God does not speak, if what he intends is not known.
5 It is necessary to indicate a substantial difference between Bataille (1986) and Girard. For the former, there is no longer sacrifice in Modernity, hence the overflow of war. For the last Girard, in turn, sacrifice is the possibility of total destruction, that is, a sacrifice of humanity as a whole, of the species as such. For McGowan (2013), the problem of Bataille's view on sacrifice is its ontology, always linked with excess and transgression.
6 On the theological dimension of Girard, see Kirwan (2009) and Williams (2000).

7 This reminds me of the work *Deadlines (literally)* by Rebecca Comay. There, the author shows how this term comes from prisoner camps in the United States civil war. She says that, in that context, they attempted to produce a physical delimitation with a strong symbolic load. This is important because, in a way, it contradicts Girard's reading – and, as we will see, Agamben's, for whom Modernity becomes a timeless *continuum*. In fact, in Girard, everything seems to come from violence; everything seems to have been already flooded by it, and what is free from it can only belong to the field of the holy life, of the mobilization of the heavenly to the earthly. We should ask at this point if precisely this religious turn in Girard is not also more nihilist than apocalyptic, since to want the mimesis with Christ, without denying the gap between him and the rest of men, doesn't it imply wanting nothing, wanting death? In sum, isn't there something more than the negation of politics, that is, the negation of the abject dimension of life? Doesn't Jesus also have his Real that divides him from Christ? Let us remember his reproach to God when he is agonizing in the cross: "My God, my God, why have you forsaken me?" (Mt. 27, p. 46).

4 *Homines sacri*

Agamben's reflection on sacrifice leads to a kind of indistinction, which nonetheless is aporetic for the subject of this book.

In his critique of the political paradigm par excellence – sovereignty – Agamben argues that all ordering criteria have today been lost. Thus, an element that was considered essential for the legitimizing discourses of the State from Hobbes onwards may no longer be active. However, this does not mean that Agamben's ideas resemble Girard's; in fact, he is far from negating politics for its incapacity to regulate violence. In his perspective, sovereignty is founded on extending the logic of abjection to erase its frontiers. Its power lies, precisely, in leaving human life to indetermination.

In this sense, sovereignty appears as a type of symbolic regulation that has been developing from Antiquity to the present. To analyze some aspects of this process, Agamben goes back to the *homo sacer*, a figure particular to Roman law. On the basis of this, he says that the present is marked by the fact that all human lives are potentially sacred, that is, sacrificeable. But this sacrifice does not refer to the old religious rituals. The "inside" and the "outside" of territoriality, the pure and the impure of customs, the norm and the exception to the law – Foucault's notion of "to make live and to let die" – are now mixed up. I should here make an essential clarification: Agamben uses an old figure related to sacrifice, but his contemporary approach to the *homo sacer* is detached from it, as I will explain later.

My intention in this chapter is to analyze in depth the "everyone" that Agamben describes. It is necessary to examine the implications of such a use of the plural (*tutti*, in Italian) as it questions the logic of abjection; that "everyone" undermines the process of distinctions and delimitations that I have sought to show from the outset. In various texts, Agamben offers the description of a context in which sovereignty shows its full foundation in the continuum of death and life, without any interruption. For this reason, it is necessary to analyze whether something is veiled in this conceptual perspective. This is imperative if we intend to assess the potentiality of thinking abjection as a figure that alludes to the lack of the political – a lack that, as I have traced with my rereading of Lacan on the Freudian uncanny, weakens the imaginary dimension and

DOI: 10.4324/9781003457022-7

the guarantee of order. To put it more clearly, it is essential to resolve how a process is sustained that is based on blurring the outlines and establishing them with no criteria, that is, how an indetermination driven by the symbolic order is sustained. Hence, it is important to consider the non-degraded, the non-abject in Agamben's argument.

To explore these issues, I will make use of the inaugural work of the saga *Homo sacer – Sovereign Power and Bare Life* [1995] – and some other texts that continued the saga – mainly *State of Exception* [2003] and, to a lesser extent, *Remnants of Auschwitz: The Witness and the Archive* [1998]. In all of them, Agamben offers the same hypothesis, although it is in the first of these books that he highlights the specificity that I use to analyze the figure of sacrifice.[1]

Agamben begins *Sovereign Power and Bare Life* by putting forward the main ideas that will structure his approach. It is very well known that Agamben often uses genealogy as a method, permitting him to pose the question about the current time and the continuity occurring over the centuries. This is undoubtedly related to Foucault's ideas and to the European world. Indeed, in the first paragraphs of *Sovereign Power and Bare Life*, he explicitly refers to the author of *The Order of Things: An Archaeology of the Human Sciences.* He does this to explain his goal of understanding modern society, situated at the point where "the species and the individual as a simple living body become what is at stake in a society's political strategies" (1998, p. 14). In this context, he uses the category of "bare life", offering a whole connection between zoe and bios, a connection noted by the Greeks centuries before and which Foucault himself thematicized with new spirit in the second half of the twentieth century. As is well known, zoe refers to life as a common attribute of living beings, while bios refers to specific forms of life.

But Agamben widens his theory by also referring to Arendt, whose contributions, he claims, must be understood within the biopolitical horizon that Foucault writes of. Agamben highlights the similarities between some of Arendt's questions and those that Foucault pursued. Thus, in a work such as *The Human Condition* [1958], Arendt understood how the decay of the public sphere is related to the rise of the private sphere, with its evident needs and sublimations that used to be restricted to the domain of the *oikos*. It is precisely in this context that Agamben locates the path he intends to follow. He states his intention to do what Foucault was unable to do due to his early death: To bring together the question about the technologies of domination and their devices of normalization with the inquiry into the "Technologies of the Self" or "the care of the self" (Foucault, 1988). In Agamben's words, to connect the "juridico-institutional models" and "the biopolitical models of power" in a reflection on contemporaneity. In this context, his hypothesis is that "it can even be said that the production of a biopolitical body is the original activity of sovereign power" (1998, p. 6). In clearer terms, Agamben writes that:

> The entry of zoe into the sphere of the polis – the politicization of bare life as such – constitutes the decisive event of modernity and signals a radical

> transformation of the political-philosophical categories of classical thought. It is even likely that if politics today seems to be passing through a lasting eclipse, this is because politics has failed to reckon with this foundational event of modernity.
>
> (1998, p. 4)

Since Aristotelian times, there have been several attempts to exclude the bare life, to the point that this "exclusion founds the city of men" (Agamben, 1998, p. 7); that is, because of it, the mechanisms unfold that make abjection something inherent to the social. However, it is an exclusion that also includes – we could call it an "inclusive-exclusion", which is none other than the pair formed by "bare life-political existence" and by "zoe-bios". In fact, as Agamben argues, all this shows that Schmitt's "friend-enemy" pair is not the fundamental concept of the political, since what is questioned is "the bare life of the citizen, the new biopolitical body of humanity" (1998, p. 9):

> The fundamental categorial pair of Western politics is not that of friend/enemy but that of bare life/political existence, zoe/bios, exclusion/inclusion. There is politics because man is the living being who, in language, separates and opposes himself to his own bare life and, at the same time, maintains himself in relation to that bare life in an inclusive exclusion.
>
> (1998, p. 8)

As I said, Agamben uses sacrifice from the very notion of *homo sacer* – "a figure of archaic Roman law in which the character of sacredness is tied for the first time to a human life as such" (1998, p. 71) – as mentioned in a passage by Festus many centuries ago:

> The sacred man is the one whom the people have judged on account of a crime. It is not permitted to sacrifice this man, yet he who kills him will not be condemned for homicide; in the first tribunitian law, in fact, it is noted that "if someone kills the one who is sacred according to the plebiscite, it will not be considered homicide". This is why it is customary for a bad or impure man to be called sacred.
>
> (Festus in Agamben, 1998, p. 71)

Thus, the *homo sacer* has an ambivalent nature:

> What defines the status of *homo sacer* is therefore not the originary ambivalence of the sacredness that is assumed to belong to him, but rather both the particular character of the double exclusion into which he is taken and the violence to which he finds himself exposed. This violence – the unsanctionable killing that, in his case, anyone may commit – is classifiable neither as sacrifice nor as homicide, neither as the execution of a condemnation to death nor as sacrilege. Subtracting itself from the sanctioned forms of both

> human and divine law, this violence opens a sphere of human action that is neither the sphere of *sacrum facere* nor that of profane action. This sphere is precisely what we are trying to understand here.
>
> (1998, p. 82)

The "bare life" is a "*[l]ife that cannot be sacrificed and yet may be killed is sacred Life*" (Agamben, 1998, p. 82; emphasis in the original). In other words, the life that is included adopts the form of an exclusion. It is a matter of the absolute possibility to receive death, a question that offers "the key by which not only the sacred texts of sovereignty but also the very codes of political power will unveil their mysteries" (1998, p. 8). This proves essential for understanding Agamben since, ultimately, his entire work discusses that of Schmitt, a thinker who is considered the true standard bearer of the discourse on sovereignty. In a clear allusion to him, he sustains a point that he would later expand on in *State of Exception*:

> Instead, the decisive fact is that, together with the process by which the exception everywhere becomes the rule, the realm of bare life – which is originally situated at the margins of the political order – gradually begins to coincide with the political realm, and exclusion and inclusion, outside and inside, bios and zoé, right and fact, enter into a zone of irreducible indistinction. At once excluding bare life from and capturing it within the political order, the state of exception actually constituted, in its very separateness, the hidden foundation on which the entire political system rested. When its borders begin to be blurred, the bare life that dwelt there frees itself in the city and becomes both subject and object of the conflicts of the political order, the one place for both the organization of State power and emancipation from it. Everything happens as if, along with the disciplinary process by which State power makes man as a living being into its own specific object, another process is set in motion that in large measure corresponds to the birth of modern democracy, in which man as a living being presents himself no longer as an object but as the subject of political power.
>
> (1998, p. 9)

By using the criticism that Benjamin (2009) leveled at Schmitt in his text on the German Baroque drama, Agamben asserts that the state of exception has become the rule. For, unlike what the controversial Schmitt expressed in his work *Political Theology: Four Chapters on the Concept of Sovereignty* [1922], Agamben argues that it is no longer a question of the delimitation of a space that puts the law at risk and which enables its realization in that same process, but a space where the law and chaos live together.[2] The state of exception as a rule includes life; to abandon it is indetermination. Hence, there is no outside of the sovereign power, no exclusion of life that has not been included, no inclusion that does not entail exclusion. We find ourselves, in any case, in the field that we have considered inherent to abjection, but with the peculiar addition that this form outlined by Agamben leads to a pure indetermination that, far from alluding to the ontological lack, suspends it. How? By generating a notable process of imaginarization, no longer in the way of Girard's last work, which suspends conflict through mimesis with Christ, through the realization of the Kingdom of Heaven on the depoliticized Earth, the negation of history and its conflictivity, but in a kind of impossibility of discernment. Is abjection then present there?

It is known that Agamben finds in the "concentration camp" an illustrative example of this process, a process that, as we have seen, escapes the spatial-temporal boundaries that articulate nineteenth-century thinking on sovereignty, for it was already under development in Roman times. However, the concentration camp does not deny the political paradigm of Modernity. On the contrary, it represents the very sign of its most extended development, which somehow seems no longer possible to exit. Thus, the ambiguity highlighted by the *homo sacer* reveals the originary structure of power that culminates in the horrors of Auschwitz and which has a particular figure in the *Muselmann* – a term used in concentration camps and masterfully described by Primo Levi in *If This Is a Man* [1947–1958]:

> This oscillation betrays reason's incapacity to identify the specific crime of Auschwitz with certainty, Auschwitz stands accused on two apparently contradictory grounds: on the one hand, of having realized the unconditional triumph of death against life; on the other, of having degraded and debased death. Neither of these charges – perhaps like every charge, which is always a genuinely legal gesture – succeed in exhausting Auschwitz's offense, in defining its case in point. It is as if there were in Auschwitz something like a Gorgon's head, which one cannot – and does not want to – see at any cost, something so unprecedented that one tries to make it comprehensible by bringing it back to categories that are both extreme and absolutely familiar: life and death, dignity and indignity. Among these categories, the true cipher of Auschwitz – the *Muselmann*, the "core of the camp", he whom "no one wants to see", and who is inscribed in every testimony as a lacuna – wavers without finding a definite position. He is truly the *larva* that our memory cannot succeed in burying, the unforgettable with whom we must reckon. In one case, he appears as the non-living, as the being whose life is not truly life; in the other, as he whose death cannot be called death, but only the production of a corpse – as the inscription of life in a dead area and, in death, of a living area. In both cases, what is called into question is the very humanity of man, since man observes the fragmentation of his privileged tie to what constitutes him as human, that is, the sacredness of death and life. The *Muselmann* is the non-human who obstinately appears as human; he is the human that cannot be told apart from the inhuman.
>
> (1999b, p. 81)

These elements are further clarified in a seminal passage in which Agamben points out that the *homo sacer* "is not the formula of a religious curse sanctioning the *unheimlich*, or the simultaneously august and vile character of a thing: it is instead the originary political formulation of the imposition of the sovereign bond" (1998, p. 85).

Thus, in denying the uncanny, Agamben fails to recognize the extimate aspect of the law; he can only highlight the effects of the indetermination produced and reproduced by the logic that has undeniably become the rule. Sometime after the publication of *Sovereign Power and Bare Life*, Agamben developed this stance in more detail in another volume of the saga *Homo sacer.* The book focuses on the measures taken by the then US president, George Bush, in light of the attacks on the World Trade Center in 2001; measures which, from his analytical thinking, express a phenomenal biopolitical display inherent to a securitist paradigm of war – not a historical break but a kind of acceleration of the process. He later expressed a similar view in explaining the origin and outcome of the health crisis caused by the COVID-19 pandemic (Agamben, 2021). All this, far from strengthening Agamben's frame of understanding of the processes, seems to enable their homogenization.

Considering these elements, it could be said that there is a strong relation between what Agamben drew attention to in 2003 and his aforementioned 1995 argument. In both cases, the figure of *homo sacer* shows that it is no longer a question of making certain living conditions possible through the law – as Schmitt intended, following Hobbes, whom he admired – but of turning the exception into the rule: "Contrary to our modern habit of representing the political realm in terms of citizens' rights, free will, and social contracts, from the point of view of sovereignty, *only bare life is authentically political*" (1988, p. 106). Precisely for this reason, Agamben claims:

> If it is true that the figure proposed by our age is that of an unsacrificeable life that has nevertheless become capable of being killed to an unprecedented degree, then the bare life of *homo sacer* concerns us in a special way. Sacredness is a line of fight still present in contemporary politics, a line that is as such moving into zones increasingly vast and dark, to the point of ultimately coinciding with the biological life itself of citizens. If today there is no longer any one clear figure of the sacred man, it is perhaps because we are all virtually *homines sacri.*
>
> (1998, p. 114)

But how can we extend this logic of abjection that seems to prolong itself limitlessly, erasing all borders? Does this itself not lead to it being debated? Or, in other words, how can we think of such an indetermination that dissolves specific and positioned forms of the *homo sacer* at the same time that it extends them?

To venture a response to such a dilemma, it is necessary to point out that Agamben does not here follow the course that Girard advocates in his reflections on the failure of sovereignty. From his perspective, sovereignty prevails and increases the power of indetermination, of killing and letting live. Thus, it feeds on crisis; it is itself crisis-made order. The fact that everyone is potentially *homines sacri* does not lead to the end of the distinctions, as Girard argued, but to their establishment within the framework of a manipulation of all types. As Chow says (2006), unlike Foucault, Agamben opts not so much for the productive side but the unproductive side of power, or even its mere, prohibitive capacity. Indeed, this turns out to be in line with a much more emphatic way of thinking of continuity than disruption or intermittence. Foucault, in contrast, focused on showing different moments of sovereignty; Agamben rather seems to de-historize the history of the *homo sacer*. Thus, biopolitics resembles thanatopolitics.[3] One could even possibly consider whether, at the core of his considerations, a kind of idea of power abuse operates that spurs a total denunciation of the political. Perhaps there is some portion of this that feeds Agamben's tendency to ignore nuances in the different configurations involved in the political pluriverse.

Whatever the reason, Agamben insists on his idea of indetermination. It is fair to say that his writing shows the insecurity of a specific form of inclusion-exclusion, which, ultimately, he decides not to fully analyze. He seemingly fails to acknowledge that if everyone is capable of being sacrificed, then who executes the ritual? Or is this a state of nature similar to what Hobbes describes, or the crudest scene of polytheism of Weber's values, where everyone is a possible perpetrator and victim at the same time? Since there is no outside of sovereignty, the Real appears entirely subsumed in the (dis)order. This would appear to be a new kind of totalitarianism – a regime that no longer acts in search of closing the gap between the public and the private (Arendt, 1976) and refers contingency to an unobjectionable ground but of imposing indetermination. In other terms, far from filling the void – as Claude Lefort (1988, 2019) notes – Agamben makes the void the true order, that is, he positivizes the lack of any order in converting it into justification, in eliminating the lack as lack.

Agamben's inquiry dispenses with Schmitt's question about subject and decision. He does not address it since he only wants to highlight that the exception has become the rule. This leads him to make a renunciation that proves very costly for his theory: Abjection is left under the rule of a judgment without explanation in the field of a kind of teleology marked by the obscurity of the *homo sacer*, thus subsuming history to the philological origin of a term that does not appear fully deployed in the political field. Consequently, as Laclau (2007) argues, Agamben's perspective leads to a kind of de-politicizing nihilism that is, nonetheless, grounded in an exaggerated politicization, a product of the actions of a faceless sovereignty:

> To be beyond any ban and any sovereignty means, simply, to be beyond politics. The myth of a fully reconciled society is what governs the (non-)

> political discourse of Agamben. And it is also what allows him to dismiss all political options in our societies and to unify them in the concentration camp as their secret destiny. Instead of deconstructing the logic of political institutions, showing areas in which forms of struggle and resistance are possible, he closes them beforehand through an essentialist unification. Political nihilism is his ultimate message.
>
> (Laclau, 2007, p. 22)

In his writings, Agamben often indicates a threat to human life, not recognizing that there is a multiplicity of forms of exclusion that are, at the same time, differentially distributed. The "everyone" of the potential sacrifice revealed by the figure of *homo sacer* is the symptom of an indetermination of something that is worth acknowledging, for, as Schmitt would say in the words of Pierre-Joseph Proudhon, "whoever invokes humanity wants to cheat" (2007, p. 54). Agamben cannot escape the infinite task of documenting forms of sacrifice that are actually not sacrifice and that fail to introduce anything new. Hence, I want to clearly put forward here the reason why order itself is full of holes, the reason why every symbolic space exists only with gaps, with processes of politicization and de-politicization that succeed each other continuously and always differently. In this context, the abject is a central element to understand the imaginary support that enables the knotting between the Real and the Symbolic, and that goes beyond the distinction between the normal and the abnormal (Canguilhem, 1978), since it shows the void that makes it possible to show the variability of such distinctions. Otherwise, as in Agamben, there is an excessive use of the imaginary register, ignoring its Symbolic-Real articulation that is always situated, always different.

Based on the above, it is possible to suggest something else: Agamben's discourse is driven by a very specific and concealed concern.

Although he positions himself as a phenomenal critic of sovereignty, Agamben seemingly only wants to attempt a mere defense of European Rule of Law, that is, a defense of the formality of a legal device that enshrined a certain type and level of life and that contributed to creating a threshold of de-politicization that characterizes the present day in northern hemisphere countries; hence his concern about Bush's measures. Consequently, it is symptomatic that when he refers to an indetermination that threatens human beings as a whole, he does not indicate the variability of abjection. In this regard, as Butler shows in *Frames of War: When Is Life Grievable?*, it is the frames of recognition that operate in the delimitation of lives that are grievable, or the themes worth addressing.[4] It is probably due to considerations like this that Agamben points out in his work on the state of exception that there is a kind of possible activity to attempt to break this borderless deployment of sovereignty. And although he does not add much about it, far from opting for the reinstatement of the liberal Rule of Law or its complete removal – as could be derived from Benjamin – in *Stasis: Civil War as a Political Paradigm*, he postulates that it is a question of interrupting the operation of the machine that leads the West toward a civil war of global scope. Thus, there would only remain the task of understanding when to interrupt the cycles of instatement and removal of sovereignty; that is to say, a kind of (a)political decision reduced to the sphere of the depoliticized individual, although without any judgment, without the chance to escape from the imaginary register, which absolutizes in indifference the aspects that constitute the complexity of politics as collective action.[5]

Some of these problems had already been noted some time before by Schmitt, or, at least, it is possible to find a good number of references in his work that allow us to understand them based on the Lacanian ontological background. In order to fully understand this controversial author in the present day, it is necessary to leave aside certain prejudices that hinder the observation of some of the most intriguing tones of his arguments. Using the figures of war and the partisan, I will show that in Schmitt there remains a chance to understand how the Real permeates the very concept that structures political life, that is, the friend-enemy relation.

Notes

1 It is surprising that, given the connection or thematic closeness, Agamben has said nothing about Girard's writing. Chow (2006) offers a possible explanation. In his view, Agamben is reluctant to accept any reading anchored in mimesis, even more so if it has a transcendent perspective, as is the case in Girard's last work. Moreover, Chow suggests that in Girard's work, sacrifice helps save some from greater violence – a possibility that is nonetheless impossible considering the human stubbornness to use increasingly more destructive violence, as indicated by the nuclear perspective. The point that Chow makes here is that in detaching the sacrificial from the *homo sacer* of the concentration camp, Agamben avoids the argument of the inevitable necessity, that is, the idea that someone had to be murdered so someone could be saved; he denies the sheer logic of the sacrificial discourse. On the other hand, neither was this Nazism's argument to legitimize its killings. This argument is relevant because ultimately Agamben points out in the *Shoah* an unrepresentable dimension, something that coincides with the indetermination that brings into play his view on politics and which escapes the term Holocaust.

2 Recall here Schmitt's famous phrase: "Sovereign is he who decides on the exception" (1988, p. 5). On the other hand, in Eric Santner's view (2005), Benjamin's idea of miracle, clearly rooted in theology, implies the idea of suspension. I speak about this Chapter 2.

3 Žižek, in contrast, offers an analogous argument between these authors: "The problem with Agamben's deployment of the notion of *Homo sacer*, however, is that it is inscribed into the line of Adorno and Horkheimer's 'dialectics of Enlightenment', or Michel Foucault's disciplinary power and biopower: the topics of human rights, democracy, rule of law, and so on, are ultimately reduced to a deceptive mask for the disciplinary mechanisms of 'biopower'

whose ultimate expression is the twentieth-century concentration camps" (2002, p. 95).

4 In this regard, see the analyses present in Hirsch and McIvor (2019) and McIvor (2016).

5 This may be linked with his approach on "inoperancy", as can be appreciated in *The Kingdom and the Glory: For a Theological Genealogy of Economy and Government* de 2007 (I thank Gonzalo Ricci for the reference).

Part Three

War

5 The Enemy

If we return to the preceding chapters, we will recall that Girard revalued the religious dimension of the social, placed sacrifice as its foundational act, and noted its capacity as an institution for the regulation of community violence. Thus, he denounced that the modern legal device generates a crisis of differences that tends to homogenize individuals. However, toward the end of his life, Girard ceased to believe in the possibility of managing violence; hence, his assessment of Clausewitz's diagnosis on the extreme nature of conflictivity as current and his rejection of any type of political mediation to control it.

From Girard's perspective, the sole desirable goal was the elimination of violence at the root – a kind of absolute eradication of all trace of it. To do so, human beings had to identify with Christ. The problem of the violent origin of the social that Modernity had attempted to conceal could then be solved definitively. In the terms I propose, it could be argued that with such a modulation implying the return of the religious and its full realization in the Symbolic, Girard ended up denying the Real in all its forms. That is to say, he proposed a kind of imaginarization of the Real by using the constituent dimension of Christ as the Real, making the Real the foundation of the social. Thus, the complexity of the Borromean knot as a grid of intelligibility disappears.

At this point in Girard's reflection, there is no room to consider abjection, the lack of grounds, and the experience of the lack in politics. Agamben, in contrast, even when he used the ancient figure of *homo sacer*, did not particularly focus on its sacrificial dimension. And although he reached a different conclusion to Girard, like Girard, he also considered excessively the Imaginary register without contemplating the nuances and aspects that make up different political experiences. For this reason, it could be said that the analytical consequences of both approaches are not entirely immeasurable despite their clear differences.

In this regard, although Agamben connected the sacred with the profane, proposing an indetermination in sovereignty, he judged that indetermination constitutive. Thus, sacrifice is ultimately stripped of its density or importance, even when Agamben himself continues to argue a kind of historical continuity in government. This means it does not necessarily appear as something

DOI: 10.4324/9781003457022-9

contradictory to modern, contemporary politics. In defense of Agamben, it has to be said that in his writing he is very careful not to compare Auschwitz with sacrifice in the Roman world, from where the primary conceptualization of Festus emerges. But it is clear that some portion of the sacrificial trail reverberates in that present that the concentration camp shed light on and brought up to date. In fact, in Agamben's view, the *homo sacer* operates over life and death, over this pair that is actually a continuum, hence its ambiguity or ambivalence. And this aspect, as I said, was present in Antiquity, to such a degree that it is the characteristic sign of the current time, unavoidable since Nazism.

For Agamben, the mark of the *homo sacer* reveals and explains the still-prevailing theological-political aspect. For that reason, life may no longer be the object that must be safeguarded and protected from the arbitrariness of power; power consists of leaving life in indetermination, in a politics of indetermination, a non-politics. As we know, Agamben saw in this the permanence of a model that makes the exception the rule, which in turn allows him to assert that social borders are erased to the point where the Real becomes an entirely manageable Real, one that can be manipulated by the Symbolic, by the extreme biopolitical paradigm that has prevailed for centuries. For this reason, it is a question of an excessive trust in the Imaginary rather than a kind of belief in the capacity of symbolization. On this point, his perspective is notably different from that of an author like Benjamin. His concern ends up being very different from Benjamin's in that he unleashes a diatribe against the trend that threatens certain legal guarantees inherent to the democratic-liberal horizon. This stance is not contradictory with the negation of the lack that corrodes every order. For Benjamin, abjection was the problem, or rather, the very existence of a lack in the Symbolic. In his view, the only possible solution consisted of suspending human order in its entirety, hence his impolitic perspective.

Agamben fails to see the Real in biopolitics; he only denounces that what appears as a problem is the key to its operation. What is interesting is that the actual exclusion-inclusion processes that he mentions could only be addressed in context and retrospectively. That is, following Agamben, there is no way to operate politically, only reactively, which takes his words to a coarse separatism with no social bond. His analytical coordinates prevent a clear view of the fact that the exclusions that enable any inclusion are always already impossible, are always already something that is linked with abjection. Under the terms I propose, Agamben fails to understand the lack and fails to contemplate a doing. The indetermination between the inside and the outside, between the norm and the exception, are expressions of the non-gap of the gap. The Lacanian approach that I propose indicates precisely the contrary: The political does not have the Real in its pocket; it always needs to deal with the Real and recreate the pocket that seeks to contain the Real, and that also constitutes it internally since there are no guarantees in its void. In this, Girard and Agamben are alike: Order – both the Christian order that must prevail and the order that must be challenged – does not leave anything out.[1]

In addressing some of the most important Schmittian thematizations in the next two chapters, I will show the social frontiers that every grouping generates and their non-sense, that is, a sense that only exists through the lack. To do this, I will begin by reviewing the grounds of the political that Schmitt sketches in the interwar period, to later connect them, in the following chapter, with his particular inquiry into the figure of the partisan. The result of this third part of the process I suggest will show the lack that corrodes and enables the very field of the political and also advance in the encounter of the metaphor of the One, with its divisions and non-relations, with which I will conclude. At this point, I would like to state that Schmitt – the "paradigmatic" thinker on sovereignty – is also the thinker who best allows us to show its failure, and not only the failure of statehood as its characteristic form, but the failure of the very field of the political. For this reason, he continues to be the thinker that has best understood failure, not from alterity but from its creativity.

It is well known that Schmitt was always sensitive to the bond between politics and war, and this aside from its undeniable influence in the context of his time. From his perspective, war reveals the complex character of social life and the tribulations of the friend-enemy distinction, key to his formulations. Like any reader of Clausewitz, he understood the problems involved in the articulation not only between order and violence but also between internal and external order. Indeed, his conceptual approach to Clausewitz's work tends to revalue the indelible political sign of every armed conflagration; hence, Schmitt considered Clausewitz a political thinker par excellence and not merely a military theoretician, a theoretician of military technology (Schmitt, 1967). This permits a broader reading that encompasses both authors, since, in some way, Schmitt observes that in Clausewitz there was already present, albeit in the making, the problem of the political leadership of the people that characterizes Modernity, namely what appears throughout his work as the problem of the decision of political unity, its articulation between the constituent dimension of power and the established authority.

Concerning the figure of the partisan specifically, which I will address in detail in the following chapter, we may recall that it always fascinated Clausewitz, as one of his most prominent commentators notes (Paret, 1985). However, in his masterpiece, Clausewitz never placed it as connected to the problem of civil war; he only detached it as part of his theorization on the defense of the territory faced with an invasion, as occurred in Spain with Napoleon's advance. In contrast, Schmitt, naturally in a different historical context, positions the partisan as the expression of the internal fracture of political unity. Without aiming to go into further detail on these aspects that link and articulate the theoretical considerations of both thinkers, I would like to point out that, in some way, Clausewitz's view allows us to question the theological-political aspect that characterized Schmitt's writing in the first years of the 1920s. In short, the partisan shows the people, and not the sovereign, as the ultimate guarantor of unity; it is, in fact, the base element that constitutes the "paradoxical trinity" of war that Clausewitz coined – a trinity that is completed with the military leader or the general and the supreme political authority. Seen from this perspective, Clausewitz's incipient theorization on the partisan becomes key to the reading, helping contemplate the importance that Schmitt would attach to it to understand the political in the second half of the twentieth century.

To thoroughly analyze war as a figure of abjection, it is necessary to note that, in *On War*, the Real of violence is not easily condensed by the political or military command. In fact, Clausewitz denies that war is a geometric, static exercise, or one in which a will can be straightforwardly imposed as if it weren't fully influenced by contingency. In Clausewitz's view, it is a complex phenomenon, rooted in society, profoundly political, but one that possesses its own nature and holds something intangible. The general, who must mediate between the people and the sphere of political decisions, faces not only the enemy on the battlefield but also, at every moment, all that he cannot control. There also exists a substantial element that reveals this and which is the spirit of war: the "moral factors" (Clausewitz von, 2007), which are very much related with what we would today call affects, that is, with a non-quantifiable element, outside of the economic register.

What is important about this is that Clausewitz makes it possible to correctly propose the symbolic task of dealing with contingency – one that is not external but constitutive of politics, and hence, of war. In this regard, Clausewitz wholly follows Niccolò Machiavelli and his view on fortune.[2] Precisely as war is always political, as is its continuation, it cannot be absolutized, turned into a pure Real. Understanding the grammar of war and the logic of politics is constituted in a theoretical-practical invocation that avoids the overflow of war or the militarization of politics. For this reason – and this is key to Schmitt's conceptualization – in war, the aim is to defeat the will of the enemy, not annihilate it:

> **War is thus an act of force to compel our enemy to do our will.**
>
> Force, to counter opposing force, equips itself with the inventions of art and science. Attached to force are certain self-imposed, imperceptible limitations hardly worth mentioning, known as international law and custom, but they scarcely weaken it. Force – that is, physical force, for moral force has no existence save as expressed in the state and the law – is thus the means of war; to impose our will on the enemy is its object. To secure that object we must render the enemy powerless; and that, in theory, is the true aim of warfare. That aim takes the place of the object, discarding It as something not actually part of war itself.
>
> (Clausewitz von, 2007, p. 13)

This passage reminds us of the aphorism: "We see, therefore, that war is not merely an act of policy but a true political instrument, a continuation of political intercourse, carried on with other means" (Clausewitz von, 2007, p. 28), a veritable dictum that has boosted its creator's fame while overshadowing the genuine study of his work (Aron, 1983). What I would like to highlight from both of these quotes is that Clausewitz, as a political and military thinker, was concerned with containing what was uncontainable, with indicating that the enemy is not something without value that must be annihilated. In this regard, his writing is far from "Total War", that is, from that conception rooted in the German militarist culture of the beginning of the twentieth century, put forward by General Erich Ludendorff (1936). Notwithstanding the above, it is undeniable that the notion of "Absolute War" that he used has often been assimilated to this view of the European interwar period, which denied political mediation and the limits of war. In other words, what appears as the hypothesis of reason in *On War* is a necessity of the era in Ludendorff, a Real that must be realized. As is known, this famous First World War soldier became a fervent supporter of Nazism, supporting a full subordination of politics to the imperatives of war, hence his estimation that all of Clausewitz's theories should be replaced. In his view, war and politics only serve for the preservation of the people, influenced by a racial life. Clausewitz never made such a consideration, despite his conservative political views.

In a well-known essay from 1930, Ernst Jünger framed the connection between war and politics in a more complex manner. He argued that both instances were being molded by a historical process of totalization. Thus, First World War only expressed a more complex and unstoppable phenomenon. The primacy of technology, which he would soon after describe in detail – more specifically in *The Worker* [1932] – cast a new tone on every dimension of social life. New conflicts saw nations exhaust their resources – material and human – at the battlefront. Everything was mobilized with the purpose of satisfying the needs of the trenches. In Jünger's view, it was not a time of the full subordination of politics to war, as Ludendorff argued, but of the subordination of life to technology:

> Still, not only attack but also defense demands extraordinary efforts, and here the world's compulsions perhaps become even clearer. Just as every life already bears the seeds of its own death, so the emergence of the great masses contains within itself a democracy of death. The era of the well-aimed shot is already behind us. Giving out the night-flight bombing order, the squadron leader no longer sees a difference between combatants and civilians, and the deadly gas cloud hovers like an elementary power over everything that lives. But the possibility of such menace is based neither on a partial nor general, but rather a *total mobilization*. It extends to the child in the cradle, who is threatened like everyone else – even more so.
>
> (Jünger, 1993:128)

In the 1932 edition of *The Concept of the Political*, Schmitt borrows the notion of "total mobilization" from his friend with the aim of showing a substantial change, primarily in the configuration of the State. This is important since it shows the extent to which Schmitt entered into a field of discussion with multiple voices. In some way, it could be said that he shared with Ludendorff the characterization of war as an existential phenomenon of community, but while still considering the substantial labor of symbolic mediation that Clausewitz supported. To such a degree that, years later during the age of nuclear deterrence, he would see in the partisan an expression of the political that questions his own conceptualization.[3]

In his most famous text, first published in 1927, Schmitt postulates that the concept inherent to the political cannot be defined by means of the State, for the State is merely a specific historical form, while the political is constitutive of existence, always elusive of attempts at circumscription to a specific institution. Hence, just like there existed specific regimes in the Greek polis and feudal authorities in the Middle Ages, Modernity managed to gestate its own political form: The Leviathan. This implies a clear orientation that nothing ensures that the State will be the final form that the political will assume in history, quite the contrary. However, even while stressing this variability, Schmitt's inquiry does not dispense with the State; it cannot precisely because his discourse is inserted in that ontological difference between the political as instituting space and politics as articulable dimension, a difference that will be central to the "Post-Foundational Political Thought" (Marchart, 2007) and, even, for a knowledge model that no longer proposes a trans-historical foundation of the social, despite the different discourses that may attempt, in theoretical or political terms, to defend a substrate or an essence. Hence, Schmitt could only think of the State understanding its modifications and imagining its possible de-structuring. So it is that in the interwar period he depicts an ontological dimension based on a change in the state form.

In his view, in the first decades of the twentieth century, the contrast of the Leviathan with bourgeois civil society hardly seemed to matter anymore, much less the compartmentalization between the different domains of culture that Weber had masterfully analyzed. In his perspective, all spheres of life seemed capable of being politicized, precisely because nothing remained outside of the political, outside of a "total State".[4] And this was essentially because all spheres of life referred to the existence of a people, to their actual lives, and it was that same existence that appeared to have been put in a trance by the global dynamics that Modernity inaugurated. In Schmitt's words:

> The equation state = politics becomes erroneous and deceptive at exactly the moment when state and society permeate each other. What had been up to that point affairs of state become thereby social matters, and, vice versa, what had been purely social matters become affairs of state – as must necessarily occur in a democratically organized unit. Heretofore ostensibly neutral domains – religion, culture, education, the economy- then cease to be neutral in the sense that they do not pertain to state and to politics. As a polemical concept against such neutralizations and depoliticalizations of

> important domains appears the total state, which potentially embraces every domain. This results in the identity of state and society. In such a state, therefore, everything is at least potentially political, and in referring to the state it is no longer possible to assert for it a specifically political characteristic.
>
> (2007, p. 22)

This was the dawn of the "total state", a political form that was prolonged over different arenas of society, nonetheless maintaining the distinction between public and private spheres. It emerged – Schmitt claims – after the crisis years of 1929–1930 and increasing government intervention in the economy, giving rise to a specific type of capitalism. In this context, also marked by the appearance of the masses in political life, Schmitt highlighted the reason why the concept of the political had its specificity. Thus, he pointed out that even though it goes beyond the moral, the aesthetic, or the economic, it can unite the heterogeneity of a society. Consequently, the political was not about other distinctions but about the friend-enemy distinction, a distinction that denotes the existential:

> The specific political distinction to which political actions and motives can be reduced is that between friend and enemy. This provides a definition in the sense of a criterion and not as an exhaustive definition or one indicative of substantial content. Insofar as it is not derived from other criteria, the antithesis of friend and enemy corresponds to the relatively independent criteria of other antitheses: good and evil in the moral sphere, beautiful and ugly in the aesthetic sphere, and so on. In any event it is independent, not in the sense of a distinct new domain, but in that it can neither be based on any one antithesis or any combination of other antitheses, nor can it be traced to these. If the antithesis of good and evil is not simply identical with that of beautiful and ugly, profitable and unprofitable, and cannot be directly reduced to the others, then the antithesis of friend and enemy must even less be confused with or mistaken for the others. The distinction of friend and enemy denotes the utmost degree of intensity of a union or separation, of an association or dissociation.
>
> (2007, p. 26)

While Socrates notes, in Plato's classical dialogue The *Republic*, that justice cannot be defined from a contrast such as the friend-enemy distinction as it is variable, in *The Concept of the Political*, that feature is elevated to the essential. Schmitt's argument should be read as a path that indicates the gap of the Symbolic – and that recovers that non-relation between the political and the State admitted from the beginning of his text – but also as an aspect that strongly highlights the hole of his own conceptualization. This brings profound consequences that should be analyzed little by little, since, for Schmitt, there is nothing of the political that refers to an essence or a principle of primary imputation. Its articulation is always contingent, as are its manifestations, so this also questions the decision on friendship and enmity:

> The criterion of the friend-and-enemy distinction in no way implies that one particular nation must forever be the friend or enemy of another specific nation or that a state of neutrality is not possible or could not be politically reasonable. As with every political concept, the neutrality concept too is subject to the ultimate presupposition of a real possibility of a friend-and-enemy grouping.
>
> (2007, p. 34)

Although Schmitt's concept of the political does not substantiate the ways in which it is manifested, it highlights its structural, symbolic nature. The enemy is also that Real that threatens the form of life itself. Seen from the outside, it is the Real of the Symbolic and the Symbolic of another field of representation. It is no coincidence that he assumes the figure of something foreign, strange to a specific community form: "He is, nevertheless, the other, the stranger; and it is sufficient for his nature that he is, in a specially intense way, existentially something different and alien, so that in the extreme case conflicts with him are possible"; hence, it can be decided neither "by a previously determined general norm nor by the judgment of a disinterested and therefore neutral third party" (2007, p. 27).

But the enemy, in Schmitt's view, enjoys political dignity. For in a world without a sovereign of sovereigns, without a supra-authority – since the Society of Nations and every such regime are, in his view, an extension of world powers – war is the ultimate political way of solving the disputes between organized units. Consequently, politics employs violence; it harbors war as one of its moments but denies the annihilation of the distinction or, to be more precise, it denies the negation of the distinction, an impolitic treatment of the political. Hence, a society must consider the truth of this perspective, and it can only do so by seeking to preserve its autonomy:

> It would be ludicrous to believe that a defenseless people has nothing but friends, and it would be a deranged calculation to suppose that the enemy could perhaps be touched by the absence of a resistance. No one thinks it possible that the world could, for example, be transformed into a condition of pure morality by the renunciation of every aesthetic or economic productivity. Even less can a people hope to bring about a purely moral or purely economic condition of humanity by evading every political decision. If a people no longer possesses the energy or the will to maintain itself in the sphere of politics, the latter will not thereby vanish from the world. Only a weak people will disappear.
>
> (2007, p. 53)

Thus, war is a moment that elucidates the political in denoting why there are always different forms of inhabiting the world, which is not a problem *per se*. Pluralism operates at the base of this perspective. For Schmitt, however, this information about reality does not mean his conceptualization is stained by militarism; the friend-enemy criterion only demands that mortal combat remain as a real possibility. Hence, he is far from assimilating what Ludendorff advocated when he denied the role of politics. For Schmitt, there is politics because the world does not exist without symbolic mediations; the world is only the world as symbolic mediation, or mediations carried out from different symbolic spaces:

> The definition of the political suggested here neither favors war nor militarism, neither imperialism nor pacifism. Nor is it an attempt to idealize the victorious war or the successful revolution as a "social ideal", since neither war nor revolution is something social or something ideal. The military battle itself is not the "continuation of politics by other means" as the famous term of Clausewitz is generally incorrectly cited. War has its own strategic, tactical, and other rules and points of view, but they all presuppose that the political decision has already been made as to who the enemy is.
>
> (2007, p. 33)

This text by Schmitt, like none other in its field, allows the thematization of the lack that corrodes the political. So far, we know that the contingency that floods the friend-enemy relation, its non-essential and hence constructed character, revalues the symbolic dimension and highlights the imaginary suture that builds unity, through alterity, thus maintaining the relevance of the impossibility inherent to the Real. However, to fully understand this last aspect, it is necessary to advance in the figure of war, even following the steps of this controversial author. To do so, it is vital to distinguish between international war and internal or civil war. "War is armed combat between organized political entities; civil war is armed combat within an organized unit" (2007, p. 32). As will be seen in the following chapter, the partisan allows Schmitt to delve into this second modality of war that is only mentioned in *The Concept of the Political*. In other words, it allows him to postulate still-untapped reflections on the evolution of the political in this other modality. Only in reaching this point will it be possible to locate the impossible and real dimension of Schmitt's conceptualization of friendship and enmity. It remains now to return to the problem of exclusion that he enshrines as structurally inevitable.

If, as Schmitt claims, every community is founded on distinction and exclusion, this does not mean that every exclusion or distinction should refer to enmity or be considered inherent to the enemy. I would like to highlight that there is a kind of distinction that questions all distinctions and exclusions, not for being first but for being abject, for emerging in the place of the lack, and hence, for shedding light on the weakness of every decision that claims to be categorical, that enables the normativity of the law, the primacy of the State. Following Schmitt, the enemy is solely a kind of "constitutive outside", whose dimension becomes key for identity, for its always precarious, specular constitution, for the gestation of a frontier that outlines an inside and an outside that are always porous. To illustrate this, it is useful to quote this long passage from *Ex Captivitate Salus: Experiences, 1945–47* [1950], an intimate text written by Schmitt during his imprisonment for his collaboration with National Socialism:

> Who is my enemy, then? Is my enemy the person who feeds me here, in the cell? He even clothes and shelters me. The cell is the clothing he donates. I ask myself, then: Who can my enemy be? To be sure, I do it in such a way as to be able to acknowledge him as enemy, and in fact it must be acknowledged that he acknowledges me as enemy. In this mutual acknowledgment of acknowledgment lies the greatness of the concept. It is not very appropriate for an age of the masses with pseudo-theological enemy myths. What is more, the theologians tend to define the enemy as something that must be destroyed. But I am a jurist, not a theologian.
>
> Whom in the world can I acknowledge as my enemy? Clearly only him who can call me into question. By recognizing him as enemy I acknowledge that he can call me into question. And who can really call me into question? Only I myself. Or my brother. The other proves to be my brother, and the brother proves to be my enemy. Adam and Eve had two sons, Cain and Abel. Thus begins the history of human kind. This is what the father of all things looks like. This is the dialectical tension that keeps world history moving, and world history has not yet ended.
>
> Take care, then, and do not speak lightly of the enemy. One categorizes oneself through one's enemy. One grades oneself through what one recognizes as hostility. The destroyers, who justify themselves by claiming that the destroyers must be destroyed, are of course bad. But all destruction is only self-destruction. The enemy, by contrast, is the other. Remember the great sentences of the philosopher: the relation in the other to itself, that is the real infinity. The negation of the negation, says the philosopher, is no neutralization, rather the real infinite depends in it. But the real infinite is the basic concept of his philosophy.
>
> "The enemy is our own question as form".
>
> Woe to him who has no friend, for his enemy will sit in judgment in him.
>
> Woe to him who has no enemy, for I will be his enemy on Judgment Day.
>
> This is the wisdom of the cell. I lose my time and win my space. Suddenly the calm that holds the meaning of the words overcomes [übereilt] me. Space [Raum] and Rome [Rom] are the same word. Wonderful are the spatial force [Raumkraft] and the germinal force [Keimkraft] of the German language. It has brought about the rhyme between word and place. It has

even preserved the spatial sense of the word rhyme [*Reim*] and allowed its poets the dark play between rhyme [*Reim*] and home [*Heimat*].

In rhyme the word seeks the filial sound of its meaning. The German rhyme is not the beacon [*Leuchtfeuer*] of the rhymes of Victor Hugo. It is echo, clothing, and decoration and at the same time a divining rod for the location of meaning. Now I am seized by the word of sibylline poets, my dissimilar friends Theodor Däubler and Konrad Weiß. The dark play of their rhymes becomes meaning and appeal.

I listen for their word, I listen and suffer and understand that I am not naked but rather clothed, and on the way to a house. I see the defenseless, rich fruit of the years, the defenseless rich fruit from which meaning springs by right [*aus der dem Recht der Sinn erwächst*].

Echo grows before each word;
like a storm from the open place
it hammers through our gate.[5]

April 1947 (2017, p. 71)

As can be seen, one's own identity is recognized and formed in the enemy. Only by interiorizing the distinction presupposed by the other is one's own choice, one's own way of life forged. To annihilate the enemy – as Schmitt claims Marxism would do to the owners of the means of production and liberalism would do with all those that do not replicate the ideals of the bourgeois world – would imply a negation of the distinction and, thus, a negation of the political itself: The enemy would thus become a disvalue.

But within a community, it is necessary to manage instances of de-politicization; spaces that enshrine heterogeneity, even when every grouping establishes an identity through differences with an other – an enemy – and presuppose a certain homogeneity – a minimum of homogeneity must exist in order to represent the Symbolic. This, to some extent, goes beyond the distinction between the existential "political" and the contextual "politics" of parties; it truly shows the importance of a de-politicization for the defense of the political and its structure of power, of hierarchies, of spaces that can be delimited within their field of action.

Many of these considerations present in *The Concept of the Political* were formulated due to the features of their own context. Indeed, Schmitt was especially concerned with the indirect powers that operated as representatives of society, breaking the unity of the political form, its aggregative instances, and not just European geopolitics with its ever-competing powers. Addressing these extreme dimensions that characterized Weimar, and always following Hobbes, whom he admired, in various texts, Schmitt maintains that the primary function of the State is to guarantee community life by canceling out civil war and repelling attacks from other States. Schmitt places this work in the constitution of the modern State of the sixteenth and seventeenth centuries, both of which were marked by bloody religious and confessional differences. Hence, just as he states, the Leviathan was formed as a veritable instrument of peace-making. However, in the times of the "total mobilization" of the first decades of the twentieth century, the State, as I have argued, underwent a substantial modification:

> The state as the decisive political entity possesses an enormous power: the possibility of waging war and thereby publicly disposing of the lives of men. The jus belli contains such a disposition. It implies a double possibility: the right to demand from its own members the readiness to die and unhesitatingly to kill enemies. The endeavor of a normal state consists above all in assuring total peace within the state and its territory. To create tranquility, security, and order and thereby establish the normal situation is the prerequisite for legal norms to be valid. Every norm presupposes a normal situation, and no norm can be valid in an entirely abnormal situation. (2007, p. 46)

From this perspective, Hobbes argued that humans reach agreements with each other, alienating their natural right to defend life with the aim of exiting the state of war of all against all, which leads to the formation of a bond of protection and obedience. When the moment of the war between Leviathans comes, the subjects can refuse to fight, since it was precisely the fear of a violent death that led them to give up their innate prerogative. But given the absolute nature of sovereignty, the State retains the power to execute those individuals who, with their disobedient actions, threaten the social contract and endanger the members of the community and society as a whole. Thus, in Hobbes (1998), there is no retraction whatsoever of sovereignty; once it exists, there is no turning back. There is only the path to empower it with spirit. But, for Schmitt, the twentieth century has overcome this problem at its root. There is no dilemma at this point.

In other words, in Schmitt's view, the "community" does not understand individuals that consider themselves outside of that community in the liberal sense, who consider themselves to be isolated beings and assert a right that is prior to politics. In this sense, the echo of certain notes of Ludendorff – or of a certain militarism – would seem to strongly resound here. For the radicalization of sovereignty that Schmitt proposes finds in the interwar period the key to making the "individual" a member of the community and not an atom that prioritizes its private interest over public interest. Thus, it is a view of the individual that differs from that of the liberal tradition that Hobbes also helped establish.

To some extent, Schmitt is thus part of typically German thinking, maybe even of Hegelian tradition, which seeks to avoid a disperse overview of the social while still assuming the heterogeneity. For this reason, in his most famous text, he argues the need to depoliticize the social to politicize the State, implying an explicit distance with Hobbes' contractarianism and a notable closeness to Emmanuel-Joseph Sieyès' notion of "constituent power". Consequently, for Schmitt, the State is born out of the decision of a people to defend their way of living and not out of the decision of individuals.[6]

Hence, it is crucial to understand the relevance of the notion of "community" [*Gemeinschaft*] in Schmitt's writing, a notion costly for the social theory of Ferdinand Tönnies (2001) and Max Weber, and for Hegel's *Elements of the Philosophy of Right* [1821] and the philosophical debate in Schmitt's own context (Losurdo, 1991). In fact, in *The Concept of the Political*, the community is affirmed in an intriguing footnote that quotes only the following words by Emil Lederer – a Jewish academic with ties to Weber – uttered during the preparations for the First World War: "We can say that on the day of mobilization the hitherto existing society was transformed into a community" (2007, p. 45).[7]

In this regard, it is interesting to observe that Schmitt neither rejects modern society from a dimension inherent to nature – on this note, he also distances himself from Romantic thinkers, as he did in 1919 in *Political Romanticism* – nor does he respond to a certain "Aristotelizing" and "neo-scholastic" hint; "Society" and "community" co-exist in tension. This can even be seen in the theological-political moment of his thinking. In *Political Theology*, Schmitt points out that Modernity inaugurates a kind of popular legitimacy that cannot be denied, despite counter-revolutionary projects like that of Juan Donoso Cortés. In this regard, nor is there an essentialist perspective of the political in Schmitt's communitarian dimension. It is as though Schmitt appeals to the community by highlighting a mythical dimension that, like every dimension of this nature, condenses the lack of the Symbolic and enables life with it, suturing it.[8]

The inherently societal construction of Modernity and that other community-oriented construction that seeks to reconnect the individual with the whole in which they live survive, though with an evident distance, which to some extent replicates the background of the problem of war. Hence the social, with its volitional, pluralist dimension, is subsumed in the hostilities to a communitarian whole that harbors it and appears as prior to it:

> In reality there exists no political society or association but only one political entity – one political community. The ever-present possibility of a friend-and-enemy grouping suffices to forge a decisive entity which transcends the mere societal-associational groupings. The political entity is something specifically different, and vis-a-vis other associations, something decisive. Were this entity to disappear, even if only potentially, then the political itself would disappear. Only as long as the essence of the political is not comprehended or not taken into consideration is it possible to place a political association pluralistically on the same level with religious, cultural, economic, or other associations and permit it to compete with these. As we shall attempt to show below, the concept of the political yields pluralistic consequences, but not in the sense that, within one and the same political

> entity, instead of the decisive friend-and-enemy grouping, a pluralism could take its place without destroying the entity and the political itself.
>
> (2007, p. 45)

The problem that Schmitt would analyze some time later, and which he would even present as *Intermediate Commentary on the Concept of the Political* [1963], is the problem that stems from this tension and its echoes within political unity. In other words, it is none other than that moment when the field of representation is fractured, that moment when every identification appears placed in a predicament. However, in doing so, Schmitt does not replicate his earlier considerations; war will never cease to be an existential opposition, he argues. The point is that he took his reflections to a certain limit point that allows me to allude to the very lack that the political entails, to a certain ontological hole that shows why frontiers are revealed as impossible within a community. The sovereign decision cannot completely turn that other into an enemy, nor portray it as a mere criminal, since there is no ground to refer to, only ground to create and recreate. There is, to put it better, pure impossibility, abjection.

Notes

1 Shouldn't orders always leave something out, precisely? How can we then think of crime or of expressions not recognizable according to the values of a community? Although the abject lacks an ontological content, its empirical dimension can not only question order from a possible resistance for its exclusions but also pose new exclusions unacceptable to life.

2 Indeed, Clausewitz von (1992) wrote an anonymous letter to Johann Fichte about his 1807 essay *On Machiavelli*, considering the formation of a national army that would free Prussia from France. In Paret's words, "The matters raised in this exchange between author and approving but also critical reader, range from basic issues of political structure and practice to an odd specific, the weapon-system best suited to meet the demands of modern war. Fichte's essay and Clausewitz's rejoinder have long been recognized as a document of Machiavelli's presence in German thought at a time when Germans reacted with conflicting assumptions and conclusions to the pressures of the French Revolution and the expansion of French power. In Clausewitz's life and work, however, his letter of 1809 was merely a segment of the long maturation of his ideas that included earlier readings of Machiavelli, a process the episode with Fichte illuminates, but did not initiate" (2015, p. 80).

3 In "*Totaler Feind, totaler Krieg, totaler Staat*" of 1937, Schmitt proposed how the concepts that gave him the title of his article were articulated. He said that it came about thanks to Clausewitz, French literature on the First World War, the Geneva conferences on disarmament, fascism, Jünger, and Ludendorff. In that context, he admitted that the "Total War" formula was very accurate, but he warned that it could well end up like those expressions that become common usage and are reduced to summary guidelines; hence his attempt to specify in what measure the war had assumed a total

dimension, aligning with a "total enmity" and a "total State". It could be argued that in Schmitt's short text, Clausewitz appears directly associated with Ludendorff and thus linked with the warmongering that Germany advocated in those years. In fact, the controversial Schmitt even seems to have subtly criticized Clausewitz when he maintained that the theory of the total war that he had mainly created was only developed with territorial disputes in mind, failing to understand naval warfare and modern aerial combat. Schmitt would later revisit such spatial topics in *Land and Sea* [1942] and *The Nomos of the Earth in the International Law of the Jus Publicum Europaeum* [1950]. It should be noted that toward the end of "*Totaler Feind, totaler Krieg, totaler Staat*", Schmitt highlights, contradicting his own concept of the political, that the worst disgrace arises when enmity stems from the conflict, as in the First World War, instead of being an authentic and total, preexisting and irrevocable enmity, inherent to the "total war".

4 A term also used by Forsthoff (1934), another renowned jurist of the time, affiliated with the National Socialist Party. On Schmitt's role in Hitler's regime, see Bendersky (1983) and Mehring (2014).

5 This is an excerpt from a poem by Theodor Däubler, "*Sang an Palermo*", included in *Hymnan Italien* of 1919.

6 This can be clearly observed in the *Constitutional Theory* of 1928.

7 For greater detail on the subject of the community as a key to reading Schmitt's thinking, see Laleff Ilieff (2020).

8 To be clear, my approach tends to negate the rigid polarity between order and exception, which is usually assigned to Schmitt's political theology, but not so much as to reject it from an indistinction, as Agamben does, but rather to problematize it in the terms of a Lacanian ontology that always assumes, on the one hand, a minimum of order, and on the other, a Real that eats away at it from the inside and from the outside. On a new reading of Schmitt's political theology, I recommend Preterossi (2022). On the problem of exception, Kalyvas (2008).

6 The Partisan

In *Theory of the Partisan*, Schmitt addresses what he didn't deal with in depth, or only mentioned, in *The Concept of the Political*, namely, the existential distinction at the very heart of the community, civil war:

> If domestic conflicts among political parties have become the sole political difference, the most extreme degree of internal political tension is thereby reached; that is, the domestic, not the foreign friend-and-enemy groupings are decisive for armed conflict. The ever present possibility of conflict must always be kept in mind. If one wants to speak of politics in the context of the primacy of internal politics, then this conflict no longer refers to war between organized nations but to civil war.
>
> (2007, p. 32)

Schmitt then shows how the political form appears weakened and threatened. Through the particular figure of the partisan, he finds an avenue of access to encapsulate this episode – hence it is, in his opinion, "the key to recognizing political reality" (2004, p. 43) of his time. The point is that although the two texts supposedly complement each other, *Theory of the Partisan* exceeds the considerations included in *The Concept of the Political*. The political in the 1963 text is founded on something more than a decision; it is founded on the lack that explains and conditions the Symbolic, and hence, the decision appears unfounded. It is here that Schmitt's theoretical-political legacy takes on another tenor that is even more relevant to the present day.[1]

This later text begins by analyzing the appearance of the partisan during the Napoleonic wars. Schmitt shows how Spanish guerrillas became the true defenders of the Iberian territory against the invasion of the French army.[2] He then outlines the most significant partisan incarnations that have appeared in the subsequent centuries. He goes through the world wars of the twentieth century, analyzes the revolutions that Marxism observed after them, and indicates their role in decolonization in Africa. However, as rich as this overview is, what Schmitt seeks to highlight is the relevance of that first appearance. It was the combatants of the peninsula who caused utter admiration and envy in

DOI: 10.4324/9781003457022-10

Clausewitz – that general who was sure that his native Prussia could not do anything similar in light of Napoleonic subjugation. But it was Clausewitz, Schmitt argues, whose famous essay on war planted the seed of a theory on the partisan, which would later be picked up and taken to its ultimate consequences by Lenin and Mao:

> In the realm of thought of these Prussian general staff officers of 1808 to 1813 there also lies the seed of the book *Vom Kriege* [*On War*], a book through which the name Clausewitz achieved a nearly mythical status. Its formula of/for "war as the continuation of politics" is the theory of the partisan in a nutshell. This logic would be taken to its limit by Lenin and Mao Tse-tung – something we still have to show later on.
>
> (2004, p. 4)

It should be noted that right down to the title of his essay, Schmidt carefully chooses the notion that he presents for his readers' consideration to continue his disquisitions on the political that he had made 30 years earlier. Seeking to avoid the technical provisions and the tactical specifications inherent to the military world, he uses the term "partisan" and not the concept "guerrilla". Schmitt takes it as read that these are not synonyms. With a similar gesture, he prevents the figure of the partisan from being reduced to the definition of a mere combat method, which could well be used by different types of players by different technical-military provisions. The point is that the concept of the partisan, unlike that of the guerrilla, appears linked to the idea of "party" to the idea of "part", thus reaffirming the crack that runs through political unity. Hence, from his view, the partisan is a figure that is inherent to the political, which alludes to the problem of the stability of order and, in the twentieth century, to the State's weakness as a specific form of unity.

In what follows, I will take the path suggested by Schmitt to analyze the ontological problem of abjection. I will attempt to highlight that, since it has a very specific inscription that is rooted in the community, the partisan undermines the established authority, showing a contradiction that can no longer be contained by the institutional channels of politics or by the ordinary mechanisms of the law, since its actions transcend the effects of the decision and shed light on every decision, emphasizing its fundamental background. Consequently, for this reading of Schmitt's work, it can no longer be simply the act of nominating and of understanding who is the subject that carries out the nomination – as is the case in *Political Theology* – but rather the hole that runs through every symbolic order, every word, that is to say, that which escapes and proves insufficient. For this reason, I will speak of the failure of the decision in terms of the impossibility of any policy, without this implying a denial of its importance, quite the contrary. Solely because of this constitutive impossibility does politics enjoy utter dignity for human affairs and is constitutive of them.

In connection with this conclusion, I will point out that although Schmitt's symbolization, which explains the political as such while allowing us to consider this failure, does not expressly assume its own failure, that is, the Real of the friend-enemy distinction.[3] In this light, it is possible to understand why this essay readdresses aspects present in some of Schmitt's earlier works. For instance, if in *The Concept of the Political* and in *Constitutional Theory* it is the people that decides its political destiny, that is, that chooses to grant itself an institutional form that will enable it to defend itself from other communities and thus become sovereign, and in *Political Theology* it is the authority's capacity for decision that stands out in order to realize the law, *Theory of the Partisan* indicates how every decision appears beset from within, from the space of representation that sustains it.

The partisan is the figure that allows us to fully understand this, since it unfolds in the hole of the political; it transits the edges of all the established legal-political categories. For this reason, in reviewing Schmitt's disquisitions, it is not only possible to understand that the political is active in the transference from the enemy to that disvalue and from the disvalue to the enemy – as Schmidt also covers in *The Tyranny of Values* [1960] – but also that this variation that politics attempts to make appears as an inherent lack that justifies it. His attempt to fix the social, then, is an attempt to stabilize a field of representation with its impossible images. We could say, provocatively referring to Lacan, that between friends and enemies there is no "sexual relation" either. In order to begin to clarify this matter, it is necessary to describe the four characteristics that Schmidt postulates to define the partisan.

The first is the partisan's as irregular combatant, that is, their confrontational actions on governmental institutions – a stance that is very well illustrated since the partisan rejects the uniform, that symbol of the established authority:

> A first touchstone was already mentioned at the very beginning of our investigation when we spoke of the partisan as an *irregular* fighter. The regular character manifests itself in the soldier's uniform, which is more than a work uniform/suit. It is a sign of his sway over the public sphere, and with the uniform he also displays his weapon. The enemy soldier in uniform is the real target of the modern partisan.
>
> (2004, p. 9)

The second alludes to the partisan's high political commitment, an aspect that Schmitt links, especially, to Marxist revolutionary parties, albeit not only these, as it is important that such a figure be rooted in a particular community, its history, and its present. Hence, he argues that the partisan has an absolute need for legitimacy if he wants to remain in the sphere of the political. Otherwise, he would become a mere criminal:[4]

> A further touchstone that imposes itself on us in present times is the intense political commitment which sets the partisan apart from other fighters. The

> intensely political character of the partisan is crucial since he has to be distinguished from the common thief and criminal, whose motives aim at private enrichment.
>
> (2004, p. 10)

The third of the characteristics that Schmitt lists is high tactical mobility – a mobility that, nonetheless, must not be merely circumscribed to the inferiority of the means of combat that separate it or distinguish it from a regular army. The methods that the partisan uses show a whole way of using technology that is significant, since they replicate an attempt to remain loyal to the search to incriminate the political decision, therefore moving along the margins, stalking with surprise attacks, from that place of the unexpected: "Agility, speed, and the sudden change of surprise attack and retreat – increased mobility, in a word – are even today a hallmark of the partisan" (2004, p. 11).

Lastly, as the fourth feature, Schmitt emphasizes the telluric nature of the partisan, his attachment to the land and the geography, an attachment that is precisely connected with the second characteristic, namely the partisan's inevitable political commitment:

> The names of Mao Tse-tung, Ho Chi Minh, and Fidel Castro, lead us to understand that the relation to the soil [*Boden*], together with the autochthonous population and the geographical specificity of the country – mountains, forest, jungle, or desert – remains undiminished to this day. The partisan is, and remains, different not only from the pirate, but also from the corsair in the way that land and sea are distinguished as (two different) elemental spaces [*Elementarräume*] of human activity and martial engagement between peoples.
>
> (2004, p. 13)

This mention of Mao Tse-Tung allows Schmitt to insert – not without fine malice – a wedge within the "real socialisms" of the time. Indeed, in doing so, he reinforces his classical judgments on Marxism, indicating the different views embodied by Russia and China on the concept of the political. As is well known, Schmitt always denounced the negation of the contingent nature of the political through the absolutization of the enemy by Marx and his followers. From his perspective, Marxism leads to the discrimination of the other; it denies the difference that enables the administration of the pluriverse of the political. Thus, it embarks on a dangerous path, for it fails to understand enmity as an element typical of the political but rather makes a form of specific enmity that drinks from the fountains of the economy into an absolute enmity. For this tradition, the bourgeois or the dominant class is deemed an other that must be annihilated. Hence, for Schmitt, Marxism denies the political in radicalizing enmity and, consequently, it seeks to neutralize and depoliticize, ignoring the always situated and specific nature of polarities.

In a famous comment on Schmitt's text analyzed in the previous chapter, Leo Strauss (1995) keenly observed that the considerations about the friend-enemy relation do not express a kind of warrior morale but a serious perspective on existence with the aim of preventing the political from lowering itself to a mere politicking or hypocritical moralism. I highlight this because Strauss' reading allows us to rethink the political in the light of an enmity that cannot be absolute, not even in a partisan form that seeks protection in its commitment to a social revolution. In this regard, Schmitt argues, Mao was closest to the essence of the political within the Marxist tradition, simply by fully understanding that every activity or praxis unfolds in a specific space, with boundaries and limits, that is, with the establishment of a theater of operations and their multiple conditionings. In turn, Lenin, the other great leader of a successful Marxist revolution, never ceased to be committed to an absolute enmity where only the revolutionary war was the true one, and all other conflagrations, expected deviations:

> Mao's revolution is fundamentally more telluric than Lenin's. The Bolshevik avant-garde, which seized power in Russia under Lenin's leadership in October 1917, is different in every way from the Chinese communists who, after a war of more than twenty years, took charge of China in 1949. The differences lie not only in the internal structure of the group but also in the relationship to the soil and the people they seized.
>
> (2007, p. 40)

In sum, by the 1960s, Schmitt seems to continue to remember what he had said some time before in discarding the humanitarian ideals of liberalism[5] and the Marxist utopia. From his perspective, the world will never be the kingdom of capitalist progress, just like it will never enjoy the absence of domination or of conflictive instances as Marx's followers intended. Liberalism and Marxism are, in Schmitt's thinking, the offspring of the modern economic paradigm that denies politics by seeking to access it only to neutralize it. They do so from moral and economic contradictions that imply an incomprehension of the friend-enemy relation. Thus, both traditions make the grave error of seeking to depoliticize the world without grasping the impossible nature of this endeavor. They do things that are utterly onerous for life in society but destined to fail. As is evident, liberalism and Marxism deny politics but use it, and in that context, they can only make the other an absolute enemy that must be discriminated against or annihilated. This is clearly an anti-political and militarist stance despite their own specific rhetoric. Schmitt addressed this at length in *The Tyranny of Values*, which is echoed, not coincidentally, in the final paragraphs of *Theory of the Partisan*, where Schmitt goes beyond the nuclear, beyond what so tormented Girard, to highlight the political dimension of technology:

> This means concretely that the supra-conventional weapon supposes the supraconventional man. It presupposes him not merely as a postulate of some remote future; it intimates his existence as an already existent reality.

> The ultimate danger lies then not so much in the living presence of the means of destruction and a premeditated meanness in man. It consists in the inevitability of a moral compulsion. Men who turn these means against others see themselves obliged/forced to annihilate their victims and objects, even morally. They have to consider the other side as entirely criminal and inhuman, as totally worthless. Otherwise, they are themselves criminal and inhuman. The logic of value and its obverse, worthlessness, unfolds its annihilating consequence, compelling ever new, ever deeper discriminations, criminalizations, and devaluations to the point of annihilating all of unworthy life [*lebensunwerten Lebens*].
>
> (2007, p. 67)

In short, in the 1960s, Schmitt returned to the subject of discrimination, which he had previously addressed in *The Concept of the Political.* However, this later work is what enables us to more clearly understand the porosity of the definitions, the limits of the existential decision, and the variations in the establishment of social boundaries. Such theoretical developments take on great importance in analyzing how Schmitt finds the other side of the revolutionary partisan in the partisan who defends the status quo, that is, in a kind of "conservative" partisan. For this, Schmitt analyzes Algeria's process of decolonization, where those who fought for independence were countered by members of the French army who adapted irregular means of counter-revolutionary action. For Schmitt, this was not merely an operational decision; the French soldiers, under the command of General Raoul Salan, fought in an improper manner for the legality of the imperialist State that they sought to sustain in Algeria. From Schmitt's perspective, a State that makes this type of action viable loses the justness of its internal demarcations and its unicity. This explains, according to Schmitt, the shift in then-President Charles de Gaulle's stance on the self-determination of African colonies, a shift which, furthermore, ultimately condemned Salan's group – *Organisation de l'Armée Secrète* (OAS) – for its criminal operations.

It could be argued that the Argentine military dictatorship of 1976, which was responsible for the disappearance of numerous citizens, was influenced by these methods that France applied not only in Algeria but also previously in Indochina. For the so-called French counter-revolutionary school, torture was considered the preferred method for countering "subversive infiltrations" aimed at altering the "correct" values of the nation. Operating in a secretive and clandestine manner, in small cells made up of members of the armed and security forces, was a necessary condition for the deployment of such repressive methods. With this, I would like to very briefly point out that what Schmitt argues in his work about the partisan – which has not been used to think the historical density of these events and their echoes in the present – allows us to specify the constitution of a process of degradation of the State as political form, as unity of a space of representation. When the State operates in a partisan manner, as in Algeria or Argentina, when it is concerned neither with social legitimacy nor with preserving its dimension of universality to manage internal distinctions, but only seeks to annihilate them, then it is no longer a State, nor does it emerge as an expression of abjection. The abject – as I have sought to show throughout this book – is the image of the lack of the Symbolic, not the negation of the lack in the Symbolic via radical discrimination. Violence is never a pure Real.

For an ontological reflection of the political, the figure of the partisan becomes crucial; it is fully related with the gestation of a space of representation and with the defense of an imaginary form of the social. The matter is of fundamental significance, for if the State judges the partisan as an expression outside of the law, then the partisan will appear as a criminal lacking the parity inherent to the friend-enemy criterion and shall be judged under criminal law.

But the partisan, as has been seen, is not merely a criminal; they are something quite different. The partisan's actions escape the confinement of words: their figure brings something extra for thinking the political, becoming a Real of state politics. Hence, if the partisans were judged emphasizing their political dimension, the State would have no choice but to admit the legitimacy of the social fracture that undermines it. Even in proclaiming them as the enemy, the partisans must be defeated with military mechanisms, elevating them to a political status that prevents their symbolic degradation. However, if this last option were to occur, the State would be reluctant to mention the qualities that Schmitt himself claimed, such as in his text in favor of the intervention of President Paul von Hindenburg during the years of the Republic of Weimar. That is to say, the State would end up abandoning any ambition of being an arbitrator of the social, becoming belligerent itself, lowering itself, like any other player, plunging the society into a chaos of a particularity that cannot be imagined as universal.[6]

This is the aporia that the very concept of the political expresses and which Schmitt makes visible, belatedly, in his 1963 text, albeit not entirely, as in order to do that it would have been necessary to possess other theoretical inputs, only available in a conceptual horizon subsequent to his, which Schmitt himself nonetheless helped forge.

In this regard, the abject nature of the partisan, their duplication as presence and absence, as authority and subject, as enemy and criminal, proposes the scopes and not only the liberties of the political definition. With this reading, however, I would not like to show an indetermination such as that seen in Agamben or propose something like the failure of sovereign mediation that Girard outlines or the negation of all decisions like the Benjamin of the *Trauerspiel*. Simply, I would like to show how the Real nests in the political, in its own ontic dimension, and in its own formulation as an explicative instance of the social.

Thus, against a reading such as Agamben's, it could be argued that there is always an outside to sovereignty that stalks its specific configuration; while faced with a perspective such as Girard's, it could be stated that it is not possible to deny such a Real by means of the construction of ideals that transcend the political, for there is no ideal whatsoever that is not questioned and that does not enable discrimination and annihilation. But, lastly, against the "canonical" Schmitt, it is necessary to recover that "Lacanian" Schmitt, which allows us to sustain that the field of the political is constituted from the lack; it is permeated by it; it is in itself unstable and impossible.[7]

To summarize, there is no way of avoiding the degradation of symbolic mediations and of the categories that sustain or explain them. Their crises refer to the recurrence of attempts to grant stability to order, to sustain instances of recognition that will never cease to introduce an other as a constitutive outside and an other – at least one – that is not an other, that is not one, that appears as something degraded, and which cannot, and must not, occupy a place in the equality of the political.[8]

Through the figure of the One, I will read the reflections of Clastres and Rancière, exploring some of the problems in the allocation of social roles and the projection of an undivided society that brings back the specular dimension inherent to the political.

Notes

1 This renders inexact and superficial the following statement by Žižek in *The Ticklish Subject: The Absent Centre of Political Ontology*: "The clearest indication of this Schmittian disavowal of the political is the primacy of external politics (relations between sovereign states) over *internal* politics (inner social antagonisms) on which he insists: is [it] not the relationship to an external Other as the Enemy a way of disavowing the internal struggle that traverses the social body? In contrast to Schmitt, a leftist position should insist on the unconditional primacy of the inherent antagonism as constitutive of the political" (2000, p. 241). However, Žižeki gets it right when, in *Welcome to the Desert of the Real!*, he points out that the Schmittian enemy is performative. Because of this, the decision is not enough.

2 "The partisan of the Spanish Guerrilla War of 1808 was the first who dared to wage irregular war against the first regular modern army. In autumn 1808, Napoleon had defeated the regular Spanish army; the real Spanish Guerrilla War began only after the defeat of the regular army. There is still no complete, documented history of the Spanish Partisan War" (2004, p. 4). On this matter, see Moreiras (2010).

3 As Palti notes, "In sum, the thinking of the political demands the desubstantialization of the subject, but once it is deprived of an identity, of any positive valence or attribute and is turned into a generic notion, merely the name of a problem, then the very concept of the political starts dissolving, becomes something vague, indefinable, and ultimately indistinguishable" (2017, p. 154).

4 In this, Schmitt could not follow Benjamin's argument in his work on violence; a criminal would never be interested in having social support to carry out their activity; it would be a contradiction.

5 See Bielefeldt (1998) and McCormick (1999).
6 I refer to *Der Hüter der Verfassung* of 1931.
7 It could be considered that in the allusion to Mao Tse-Tung (2007), in a work whose subject is the partisan, there is a more or less explicit use of the "one" that is divided into "two" and which, according to Mao, leads to the contradiction inherent to dialectics. However, the reading I suggest on Schmitt's ideas makes of the "two" – the partisan – that denies the "One" – the State, the political unity or community – a "non-two", which threatens a "non-One". I will revisit this issue in the last section of this essay.
8 Thus, returning to Žižek, it can now be said that the Schmittian partisan notes that "the appearance which conceals the fact that, beneath the phenomena, there is nothing to conceal" (2000, p. 198), but, precisely because of this, because there is nothing, there is always something that needs to articulate that lack.

Part Four

The One

7 Being *pané*

It is easy to observe the importance of the figure of the "One" in different episodes of the tradition of Western thinking. Perhaps one of the most relevant was the publication of *Discourse on Voluntary Servitude* – in French, *Discours de la servitude volontaire ou le Contr'un* [1548][1]– by Étienne de La Boétie, a fundamental text not only for the Monarchomach challenge present in the anonymous *Vindiciae contra tyrannos* [1579] but also for certain theoretical and political appropriations long after the fact in relation to, to a great extent, anarchism, socialism, and the challenge of totalitarianism, as well as anarcho-capitalism. It could even be said that the theme of the "One" associated with domination has not ceased to permeate related debates of utter relevance and permanence, such as, for instance, those related to populism and its connection with democracy. Argentine thinkers have done a vast amount of work in this regard due to the populist democratizing experiences – such as the movements under Yrigoyen and Perón – that unfolded in the first half of the twentieth century. Thus, populism may not be the condensation of the One of domination as in Europe, but a different way of thinking about political unity beyond the meaning prevalent in much of the Western world.[2]

In this chapter, I will use the figure of the "One" in a much more limited manner. It will suffice for me to simply use its most primary meaning, that is, a certain undivided dimension of political order. Thus, the One will be understood as a metaphor that alludes to the imaginary closing of the social; to that aspect that enables the formation of an identity beyond the multiple aspects that constitute it. This is, then, a use that seeks less to understand the loss of freedom at the hands of a rigid power center than the necessary but impossible closing of a heterogeneous field, that is, one that leads to the establishment of identity boundaries.

I barely remember what I have said up to this point, but it is evident that the criticisms that Girard and Agamben made of the paradigm of sovereignty made it possible to address the problem of war, distinguishing a "constitutive outside" – an alterity – from those instances that appear discriminated, displaced, or on its inside. Thus, I have been able to address Schmitt's disquisitions on the political, seeking to understand the circumstances of decision:

DOI: 10.4324/9781003457022-12

the circumstances that the action of nominating enables for social life, its deployment in war, and its actions in the criminal. Far from considering these dimensions as abominable, I strove to understand them as inherent to the symbolic field. With the specific use of the partisan that Schmitt developed in the 1960s, I was able to then focus on how the Real permeates the field of the political itself. In this context, the reversibility of the friend-enemy category showed the gap that constitutes the Symbolic. From my perspective, the partisan reveals the abject in that it is that image that alludes to the lack, to the uncanny dimension noted by psychoanalysis, to the imaginary component that enables the knotting between the registers of reality, just as Lacan indicated in his unpublished seminar *RSI* [1974–1975]. As "semblance of Real", the partisan has a Symbolic inscription that allows us to precisely understand it as the abject.

I will now take Clastres and Rancière as references in order to observe how their critique of sovereignty allows us to consider this same aspect from another perspective. Unlike Girard and Agamben, both thinkers were always far from inquiring into the forms of social regulation of violence; they really sought to denounce all social regulation, all dominance. Drawing from their considerations, I will address certain aspects that refer to the space of political unification as an unavoidable element, an element that enables identity, or, to put it another way, an element without which no identity is possible. Nonetheless, I will aim to show that their respective disquisitions were put forward from very different positions and conceptual frameworks. Indeed, the figure of the One does not appear in the same manner in each bibliographic corpus; in Clastres, there is an explicit use of this term, while in Rancière, it is a kind of figure by means of which it is possible to ground his invectives against the consensualist schemes of the political. On the basis of this, it is possible to understand why Clastres used the legacy of Étienne de la Boétie, inscribing himself in it to then deny all domination, even more so domination by the modern sovereignty that arose in Europe, while Rancière found the fundamental problem in the gestation of a specific "distribution of the sensible", which allocates social roles and denies the fiction of unicity. Clastres proposed an accurate contradiction between life in Europe and its obverse – certain indigenous communities of South America – while Rancière focused on the characteristic dynamics of every political order, regardless of their history.

In short, Clastres rejected the One of sovereignty, praising the One of community, while Rancière denounced every form of the One since it referred to the homogenization and the negation of conflict.

At this point, the relevance of the One in addressing abjection begins to be established. With this, I would like to emphasize here, as a theory, that if there is One, it is because there is an other – or something that struggles to be recognized – which it is not, but also an other that is, in the same way, One. The value of this statement, however, lies in observing that just as any unification between two ones is impossible, every one also has its gap, its internal dislocation.

To develop this argument, I will refer to two works by Clastres: *Society Against the State* [1974] and *Archeology of Violence* [1977]. Given the subject of each and their closeness in time, I will analyze them jointly. They are in fact related writings, the product of Clastres' field research with the Aché, Guarani, and Yanomami communities of South America. I am interested in highlighting how Clastres used these forms of life to criticize the evolutionism of certain anthropological approaches, mainly those following the normativism of Émile Durkheim and of Marxist economicism. Thus, Clastres emphasizes with his research that the course taken by so-called primitive societies is very different to that of the Western nations and that there is nothing that leads the social to a specific state or destiny; societies – he claims – can lack domination. Those communities that do not know the State are not incomplete or underdeveloped; they are communities that express a struggle against the State, against the emergence of the "One" that is represented as the holder of sovereignty and which fragments the community body into the dominating and the dominated.

It is clear that with such a perspective, Clastres expresses a somewhat anarchist view that he seeks to justify. But this is not the main point that concerns me. What is significant is that his perspective does not deny the relevance of politics, or, more accurately, the political nature that necessarily occurs in the social. Indeed, the author highlights this feature throughout his work to such an extent that, with this, he seeks to portray a different mode of the political to the one developed by the paradigm of sovereignty. Unlike Girard, Clastres' anthropology does not seek a transcendental dimension to be realized but to show a correct organization of the social that has already occurred, present still as vestige, which modern evolutionism and imperialism denied. However, Clastres says nothing about the origin of this model that must be de-structured; rather, he challenges it entirely, considers it known, and takes it for granted; he only focuses on explaining the true and non-inverted image of the social.

Following this goal, in his two most renowned texts, he attempts to avoid the divorce that occurs within sovereignty, that is, the fold that distinguishes men and women by their effective power, by the possibility to impose their will. Hence, he explicitly recovers the spirit of La Boétie's text. In this line, he says something fundamental for his constant argument with Marxist tradition: Social organization is not reduced to the verdicts of the economic; what happens in production relies on a specific configuration of the political:

> Society's major division, the division that is the basis for all the others, including no doubt the division of labor, is the new vertical ordering of things between a base and a summit; it is the great political cleavage between those who hold the force, be it military or religious, and those subject to that force. The political relation of power precedes and founds the economic relation of exploitation. Alienation is political before it is economic; power precedes

> labor; the economic derives from the political; the emergence of the State determines the advent of classes.
>
> (1989, p. 198)

In short, Clastres views power as the heart of the social. Thus, in primitive societies, power does not bear a relation to its diachronic dimension, to succession or inheritance – which distances him so much from Benjamin's concern over deposition and the instauration of the law as well as from Weber's perspective on types of legitimacy – but to its synchronic dimension. Clastres identifies a risk, namely, that the community's power yields to the domination of a One. If this occurs, the One will appear as external to society, and the model inherent to Europe will be founded, which will in turn cause violence to be tied to domination. In this regard, unlike Girard, Clastres considers that the problem is that this alliance occurs, for although archaic societies are not societies without violence – they are actually societies for war – they are societies without domination: "An image dominant enough to induce a sociological observation: primitive societies are violent societies: their social being is a being-for-war" (1994, p. 140).[3]

In noting this feature, Clastres is compelled to distinguish his analytical approach from the Hobbesian, with its classical thematization that likens "state of nature" to "state of war". In his view, war is neither the other of the social nor the product of its defection; nor is it the One that enables the constitution of life in community. For Clastres, there are different forms of social organization that locate war and violence in very different places. His approach favors those forms of political life that deny domination and not those others that present it as something given or inevitable, even inexorably tied to violence, monopolizing it in an institution. Thus, he seeks to argue with the most important anthropological discourses of the time that explain why war occurs in primitive societies. He highlights the three major stances with which he intends to argue.

First, Clastres refers to the "naturalist" perspective, which stresses that primitive societies are not societies for war but societies where the war logic prevails due to the power of the hunter group. From this approach, there would exist a social differentiation that is guaranteed and sheltered by the power of weapons. Instead, Clastres advocates that war implies an aggressiveness that hunting does not have, and therefore there is confusion. The naturalist stance cannot outline the complete foundation of the war moment in societies without domination.

Second, Clastres argues with the "economicist" perspective of anthropology, which understands war as a consequence of the scarcity inherent to all subsistence economies. To counter this hypothesis, Clastres argues that Aché society has a subsistence economy that is, in fact, an economy of abundance, so much so that its members work only the necessary amount and spend the rest of the day at leisure. In this context, Clastres highlights that this has not always been the case and that not all Indigenous communities of South America have or had the same structure. The communities that were tied or assimilated to the Inca Empire had to pay burdensome taxes, which required constant, exhausting productive labor.

Third and last of all, Clastres opposes the perspective of his admired Claude Lévi-Strauss, more specifically, the perspective that sees war as an expression of a failed exchange. According to Clastres, this perspective – dominant in the anthropology of his time – understands primitive societies not as societies for war but as societies for exchange. Thus, only on certain occasions are they forced to resort to and use weapons to gain control or possession of the different materials and goods that the flow of trade cannot guarantee. The main problem that Clastres notes in this reading is that violence is left without explanation. In his view, violence is not an effect of trade or unsuccessful exchange; on the contrary, the exchange that primitive societies carry out finds its raison d'être in war needs. This type of society trades with others with the aim of reaching agreements that may allow them to wage war. Alliances are thus essential, not only for moving across foreign territories with relative security and protection but also to ensure that one's own population is not attacked in betrayal and does not suffer from its defenselessness when their men are occupied with the war campaign.

In conclusion, in Clastres' view, war expresses the independence or autonomy of the Stateless society. However, he clarifies that war does not offer the possibility of the emergence of the political in terms of the friend-enemy relation: War is the modality that the primitive society adopts, the element that allows its internal homogeneity and its external distinction. The violence that drives it appears at the service of a frontier that is established between the society and its outside. As Clastres notes in *Archeology of Violence*:

> What is the function of primitive war? To assure the permanence of the dispersion, the parceling, the atomization of the groups. Primitive War is the work of a *centrifugal logic*, a logic of separation, which is expressed from time to time in armed conflict. War serves to maintain each community's political independence. As long as there is war, there is autonomy: this is why war cannot cease, why it is permanent. War is the privileged mode of existence of primitive society, made up of equal, free and independent sociopolitical units: if enemies did not exist, they would have to be invented.
>
> (1994, p. 164)

Thus, Clastres is not that far from the Schmittian perspective, even when, in his view, Schmitt established an improper type of political unity, inherent to domination. However, and unlike Schmitt, Clastres sees war not as a possibility but as a necessity to be satisfied daily in order to sustain the unity of society, to sustain its belligerent way of being. What is interesting about this is that the negation of the One of sovereignty that Clastres advocates through the recovery of the State-less society has its counterpart in the upholding of the One of non-domination, of a specific type of community, faced with other forms of community, which are potentially enemies:

> What is the State? It is the total sign of division in society, in that it is a separate organ of political power: society is henceforth divided into those who exercise power and those who submit to it. Society is no longer an undivided. We, a single totality, but a fragmented body, a heterogeneous social being. Social division and the emergence of the State are the death of primitive society. So that the community might assert its difference, it has to be undivided: its will to be a totality exclusive of others rests on the refusal of social division: in order to think of themselves as We exclusive of Others, the We must be a homogeneous social body.
>
> (1994, p. 165)

In the following prophetic story of the Guarani people – included in *Society Against the State* – this One of primitive societies is precisely observed from a cosmological justification:

> One is everything corruptible. The mode of existence of the One is the transitory, the fleeting, the ephemeral. Whatever is born, grows, and develops only in order to perish will be called the One. What does that mean? Here one gains access, via a bizarre use of the identity principle, to the foundation of the Guarani religious universe. Cast on the side of the corruptible, the One becomes the sign of the Finite. The world of men harbors nothing but imperfection, decay, and ugliness: the ugly land, the other name for the evil land. *Ywy mbo'e megua*; it is the kingdom of death.
>
> It can be said – Guarani thought says – that everything in motion along a trajectory, every mortal thing, is one. The One: the anchorage of death. Death: the fate of what is one. Why are the things that make up the imperfect world mortal? Because they are finite; because they are *incomplete*. What is corruptible dies of unfulfillment; the One describes what is incomplete.
>
> (1989, p. 172)

Following what Clastres postulates, it could be said that the society with the State is the One that denies the community; the Stateless society is a kind of non-One; it is the true totality without the duality that enables domination, which is none other than asserting that the community is the true One that abjures submission. This leaves the inquiry precisely at the point at which I would like to explore now to understand the internal organization of this class of grouping that Clastres investigated.

It seems that Clastres does not take into account that the social differentiation that occurs in primitive societies may not entail the political form of domination, but it clearly represents a type of domination that leads to the problem of abjection, that is, to a One that only admits certain forms of symbolic inscription that homogenize the field of representation, thus denying its intrinsic lack. I will take two examples from *Society Against the State* to illustrate this issue: two examples taken from the Aché community that refer to different forms of the cursed to forms of being in a *pané* state (1989, p. 108). Only one of them, however, will reveal the place of the abject that can be located in Clastres' approach. The contrast between the two examples will be both useful and necessary.

The first of these examples refers to Chachubutawachugi, a widower, excluded from using the bow and arrow due to his lack of hunting skills, rejected by the women of the community, and constantly mocked by the children. The second looks at Krembegi, a homosexual who behaves, dresses, and sings like the women of the group and who even does the same gathering work as them. This is a member that has sexual relations with other men without the community punishing him or looking down on him.

Chachubutawachugi lives in solitude; excluded from the symbolic masculine field, he inhabits an uncomfortable area between the bow and the basket due to the prevailing sexual division of labor. In this context, he has no choice but to hunt for food every day using his own means and to participate in the religious rituals with his own singing style. Krembegi, in contrast, appears to be accepted in the order of the basket and included in the women's work: He uses the female semblant to be harbored by the community. For this reason, the two modalities of being in a *pané* state that Clastres describes do not imply the same in political terms; do not question the Symbolic and its knotting with the Real and the Imaginary in the same way; in fact, neither are they harbored in the same manner by the community:

> The Aché maintained a quite different attitude towards each of the two basket carriers mentioned above. The first, Chachubutawachugi, was the butt of general ridicule, albeit free of real meanness. The men made light of him more or less openly, the women laughed behind his back, and the children respected him much less than the rest of the adults. Krembegi on the contrary attracted no special attention; his ineptness as a hunter and his homosexuality were deemed evident and taken for granted. Now and then certain hunters would make him their sexual partner, displaying in these erotic games more bawdiness – it would seem – than perversion. But this never resulted in any feeling of scorn for him on their part.
>
> (1989, p. 109)

The first of these cases expresses a degraded life; it shows what must be excluded, though not necessarily expelled from the community. Thus, the existence of Chachubutawachugi serves as a collective amalgam, as a true example of men's behavior. To some extent, it is an expression of what Butler would call "queer".

In the second of the cases, although Clastres shows how the community puts a strong symbolic consideration on Krembegi's way of being, his life appears as an expression of social order, or even as an irrelevant expression for the correct development of the social. Krembegi is a difference that does not alter order; he appears already included as an exception to the rule, though not as an exception of the Symbolic as such; hence, he does not represent a problem or a threat; consequently, it is not the abject expression that reveals the ontological gap. Chachubutawachugi, in contrast, is the abject of the Aché community. With all his particularities, with the rejection of the dominant masculinity, with his refusal to be inscribed, as a counterpart in the order of the "basket", he stands in the empty space, in that place where meaning and foundation collapse. It would be a most evident simplification if we said that he is a mere "deviated" case, for what we could consider "deviated" is merely the sign of the impossibility of orienting Chachubutawachugi; it is his radical discomfort because he cannot be assumed to be deviated by the order. Chachubutawachugi is the abject that is *pané*.

Clastres fails to notice this because, in a way, Chachubutawachugi is the Real of the image that Clastres praises in the organization of the society against the State. Chachubutawachugi represents the most severe internal threat to the community, and not because he is a conspirator or a traitor, but because he expresses the meaninglessness of the political order, the activity that always creates the symbolic, and is therefore violent. In fact, it is interesting that Clastres admits that this is a member who does not find his place anywhere and that his situation is much more uncomfortable than that of Krembegi:

> Chachubutawachugi, on the other hand, constituted in his very person a kind of logical scandal. Because he was not situated in any clearly defined place, he evaded the system and introduced an element of disorder into it: from a certain viewpoint it could be said that the abnormal was none other than he. Whence too, more than likely, the psychological difficulties he was experiencing, and an acute feeling of abandonment: that is how difficult it is to maintain the absurd conjunction of a man and a basket. Pathetically, Chachubutawachugi tried to remain a man without being a hunter: he thus lay himself open to ridicule and jeers, for he was the point of contact between two areas that are normally separate.
>
> It is logical to assume that these two men preserved with respect to their baskets the difference in the relationship they entertained with their masculinity. As a matter of fact, Krembegi carried his basket like the women, that is, with the headband round his forehead. As for Chachubutawachugi, he passed the same bandeau round his chest and never round his forehead. This was a notoriously uncomfortable way of carrying a basket, more tiring than any other; but for him it was also the only means of showing that, even without a bow, he was still a man.
>
> (1989, p. 110)

In Clastres' description, there is no problematization of these cases related to the topic of domination. The undivided community manages everyday life, seeking to block this type of situation so that the supposed non-domination is sustained. But Chachubutawachugi questions something more than domination; he questions that point where the political and the impolitic seem to blur; he expresses the lack that must be recreated, symbolized, in some way. Clastres, who converts his aversion to the One of sovereignty into a praise of the One of society, does not recognize other means of domination that continuously inform politics and verify the treatment that politics gives to the Real. Hence, he merely highlights that in primitive societies there is no break in the order unless it is through the action of another community that seeks to conquer it, perhaps a society with a State, one of Christian origin, or a society strongly organized to collect taxes of Indigenous origin.

It is interesting to note that in his research Clastres indicates that the military chief and the political chief of the Community One occupy a highly defined place that they will never be able to fully use to become truly dominant over their fellow people. The military chief is only a warrior who cannot wage a war motivated by private ends, while the political chief plays an apparently privileged role as the only polygamous person, but he is completely tied to the service to the community. Indeed, he must secure the group's harmony, be generous with others, respond to members' infinite demands, make gifts to please them, and master the art of public speaking. This last aspect is key: The political leader must *speak well*. His use of language, unlike that of the One of sovereignty and unlike the figure of the charismatic leader who "charms" the masses, is not a sign of power or a source of legitimacy. Clastres emphasizes that it is the community that is responsible for making sure that "word" and "power" never meet. Thus, the leader appears fenced off by the community, fenced off by his women, forced to speak well, forced to play a role as constant as it is exhausting, for beyond his qualities as speaker, no one ever hears what he says; everyone pretends not to pay attention to him, not to hear him, and yet they are still controlling him. A cruel game that the whole community plays, forcing their chief to an infinite speech to restrain him, to ensure non-domination:

> What does the chief say? What is the word of a chief like? First of all, it is a ritualized act. Almost without exception, the leader addresses the group daily, at daybreak and at dusk. Stretched out in his hammock or seated next to his fire, he delivers the expected discourse in a loud voice. And his voice certainly needs to be strong in order to make itself heard. As a matter of fact, there is no gathering around the chief when he speaks, no hush falls, everybody goes about their business as if nothing was happening. The word of the chief is not spoken in order to be listened to. A paradox: nobody pays attention to the discourse of the chief. Or rather, they feign a lack of attention. If the chief, by definition, must submit to the obligation to speak, the people he addresses, on the other hand, are obligated only to appear not to hear him.
>
> In a sense, they lose nothing in the bargain. Why? Because the chief, for all his prolixity, literally says nothing. His discourse basically consists

> of a celebration, repeated many times, of the norms of traditional life: "Our ancestors got on well living as they lived. Let us follow their example and in this way, we will lead a peaceful existence together". That is just about what the discourse of a chief boils down to. One understands why those for whom it is intended are not overly disturbed by it.
>
> (1989, p. 153)

This lack of attention from the community shows the undivided role of the social that Clastres seeks to reaffirm in his crusade against the paradigm of sovereignty. It is a lack of attention that is feigned but sustained as a way of being that seeks immunity from dissuasion and change. The community shows its solvency by refusing to be tempted and not succumbing to that which can emerge and disrupt its way of life. And in doing so, Clastres' archaic society is utterly conscious; only in this way can it ensure its existence in a world of domination. Words do not convince. The community comes up every day against that which stalks it from within, and, in defeating it, it shows all its power. Hence, the political leader can only deal with the old stories and their ancestors' vicissitudes. Thus, he shows that tradition dominates him, that *it speaks to him*, that his word is entirely of the Other, and not that he dominates tradition and that he can make use of the Other to rule over his peers. His speech will never be stronger than the customs, which are already solid; his art will never be enough to bring in a different way of doing or being. There is no one individual that can sign off such communitarian, homogeneous, condensed space. The rhetoric of the political chief becomes the sign of all the power that he lacks; it is an empty discourse. For this reason, both leaders of the community will never be the One and will never be able to conspire together guided by secret ambitions:

> It is in the nature of primitive society to know that violence is the essence of power. Deeply rooted in that knowledge is the concern to constantly keep power apart from the institution of power, command apart from the chief. And it is the very domain of speech that ensures the separation and draws the dividing line. By compelling the chief to move about in the area of speech alone, that is, the opposite of violence, the tribe makes certain that all things will remain in their place, that the axis of power will turn back exclusively to the social body, and that no displacement of forces will come to upset the social order. The chief's obligation to speak, that steady flow of empty speech that he owes the tribe, is his infinite debt, the guarantee that prevents the man of speech from becoming a man of power.
>
> (1989, p. 154)

As Clastres says at the end of *Archeology of Violence*, the archaic society "repeats Hobbes' discourse by reversing it: it proclaims that the machine of dispersion functions against the machine of unification: it tells us that war is against the State" (1994:167); hence, "it is said that the history of peoples who have a history is the history of class struggle. It might be said, with at least as much truthfulness, that the history of peoples without history is the history of their struggle against the State" (1989, p. 208). However, none of this removes internal domination, the symbolic imperatives that shape the social.

Faced with Clastres' undivided One, it is possible to mobilize Rancière's words and understand that every allocation of social roles comes from a logic attentive to the fixations that persist in denying their own internal division.

Notes

1 English editions do not tend to include the second part of the title, which could be translated in its entirety as "Discourse on Voluntary Servitude or Against the One".
2 This can be seen in the debates prompted by Laclau's formulations present in *On Populist Reason* [2005].
3 This consideration has as its principle and horizon the configuration of power in Europe and, from there, in all its areas of influence. The variation on the "One" – a metaphor that is rooted in the confessional struggles of the beginning of Modernity – is inscribed, precisely, in a difference that seeks to invert the place where the burden of the pathological falls.

8 The Part of Those That Have No Part

In *Disagreement: Politics and Philosophy* [1995], Rancière maintains that any view that values the undivided aspect of a community conceals a constitutive imbalance. Every hierarchy, every label, and every allocation of social roles is permeated by a calculation that cannot turn out well. And this is not because of a misuse of mathematics, but because at the heart of the social, there operates an irreducible disagreement, a Real that alludes precisely to the discursive practice of the social. Hence, "disagreement occurs wherever contention over what speaking means constitutes the very rationality of the speech situation". Thus, "the interlocutors both understand and do not understand the same thing by the same words" (1999, p. xi). To put it more clearly:

> Disagreement is not the conflict between one who says white and another who says black. It is the conflict between one who says white and another who also says white but does not understand the same thing by it or does not understand that the other is saying the same thing in the name of whiteness. The term is so broad it obviously calls for a certain amount of fine-tuning and obliges us to make certain distinctions. Disagreement is not misconstruction. The concept of misconstruction supposes that one or other or both of the interlocutors do or does not know what they are saying or what the other is saying, either through the effects of simple ignorance, studied dissimulation, or inherent delusion. Nor is disagreement some kind of misunderstanding stemming from the imprecise nature of words.
>
> (1999, p. x)

Consequently, the social space appears as an eminently discursive space permeated by an inconsistency, a hole. The Real in the Symbolic and the Real as limit to the Symbolic clearly emerge here in Rancière's work. Thus, he not only highlights the point where the Imaginary and the Symbolic converge, and which tangentially touches the status of the Real, but also warns about the constitution of the communitarian field.

However, the problem of disagreement is far from related to the differences in the degree of rationality of speaking beings. What Rancière truly values

DOI: 10.4324/9781003457022-13

throughout his work is precisely the equality of intelligences; his emblematic work *The Ignorant Schoolmaster: Five Lessons in Intellectual Emancipation* [1987] shows this. In 1995, Rancière keenly shows something else: How disagreement is presented in the form of a distortion, an offense against the intentions that seek to negate the fissures and conflicts that occur in the social space. The "One" of community, supposedly undivided, is beset by a Real that corrodes it internally. Hence, Rancière directly attacks those theoretical paradigms – such as consensualist ones – that argue that the social cannot be stained by conflict.

Recall that the symbolic order seeks to speak out above any noise that affects a specific ethical provision and any given normative perspective. Thus, it attempts to reallocate places and think of the matrix that defines roles and preferences. However, as Rancière writes, none of this can work – not at least in the intended sense, not at least once and for all. Rancière is more concerned with seeing the fault in the productivity of power rather than highlighting its structuring effects, perhaps as can be drawn from a light reading of Foucault's courses. The point to highlight, then, is that all distribution of the sensible is beset by this ontological matter. In addition, recall that if the cases of disagreement refer to the use of words, what is then shown is an inherent political nature, a necessary articulation between word and power, that which Clastres was able to divorce in his research into the "societies against the State". In order to clearly state the value of such considerations, Rancière goes back to the Greek perspective.

In his view, in the Aristotelian disquisitions, the *Logos* that distinguishes men from beasts appears as the guarantor of the social bond and of the possibility of an ethical horizon. In fact, in Aristotle's *Politics*, life is not just about the satisfaction of biological needs but also about happiness, which does not exist without a public inscription, for the Greek world is not the Modern world; hence, it was not possible to think of happiness from the individual. Rancière, however, points out that Aristotle's attempt to harmonize the sensible implies a negation of the disagreement, a "partition of what is common" (1999, p. 5). The parts of the *polis* that Aristotle analyzes appear connected by their distinctions, which can, in turn, be rearticulated for the sake of the "common good".

It could be said that Rancière offers a reading of Aristotle's work that indicates a difference with Plato's. While in the *Republic* Plato seeks the formation of a *polis* without conflict, in *Politics,* his disciple assumes its irreducible character, and hence the need for the political regime to manage its emergences or community crystallizations. From this alone, it is possible to understand the different levels of analysis that Aristotle suggests regarding monarchy, aristocracy, and the republic, three forms of government that are equally fair and which pursue the common good. Indeed, the "republic" is the regime that Aristotle values the most, precisely because of its capacity to articulate instances that enable the involvement of the wealthy and the poor – the main parties of the *polis* – by means of a certain mixture of mechanisms of oligarchy and democracy – both deviated regimes, for they only pursue the specific well-being of the ruling sector.

What I want to highlight is that Rancière argues how Aristotle distinguishes three "parts" of the *polis* with their respective assets. Thus, wealth belongs to oligarchy, virtue belongs to aristocracy, and freedom belongs to democracy. For Rancière, this is an attempt by Aristotle to harmonize what is inscribed in disagreement. In this sense, it is not that Aristotle understands harmony wrongly; it is rather that he does not entirely assume its impossibility, its utopian dimension. To put it clearly, any harmony advocated by a discourse that seeks to be dominant is doomed to failure, precisely because harmony is not possible in the political; the political exists because of an ontological lack that is impossible to solve.

The "parts" do not exist, or exist only as a condition of an inaugural act; the outlined parts are not therefore quantifiable or definable; they are not parts at all, much less do they have an intrinsic or direct relation with their allocated attributes. Rather, this (non)relation comes from the act itself of nominating and symbolizing, for there is nothing outside of language. In other words, politics exists because there is a gap in the community that cannot be closed and which is verified in the symptom – a symptom that is nothing but the result of the actions of the Symbolic over the Real. In this sense, Rancière notes that "[t]here is politics – and not just domination – because there is a wrong count of the parts of the whole" (1999, p. 10).

With this description, Rancière notes that democracy lacks its own asset, for if the freedom of the *demos* is the freedom of the public, the public is not the property of any one sector. Here is the blind spot in Aristotle's argument. But Rancière also remarks that no other political configuration aims to be as extensive in its scope as democracy. Thus, the outlined part of the *demos* that Aristotle indicates is a part that has no part.

It could be said that, in Rancière's view, there is no political model or paradigm that fits the Real because the Real limits every model; it fractures every allocation. This is compatible with the premises of Lacanian non-ontology and my reading on the abject as an expression that emerges in the place of the lack, expressing an impossible Real that undermines the knotting of every symbolic configuration; hence its consideration as a semblance of the Real.

Continuing with Rancière, his analysis of the Greek model enables him to highlight that there is always an allocated part that has no part. The "part of those that have no part" is made up by those who are not entirely excluded from the social, although they are subordinated, left as objects in the field of representation, whose dominant players have already defined proper conducts and established ethical expectations. In other words, those that have no part are nothing without the Symbolic; they are not outside of history. Rather, they are that unwanted effect. Hence, although the task of identifying and inscribing the players and the processes in a specific field appears as necessary, it is a failed endeavor. Consequently, from the point of view that I put forward, it is less a matter of thinking of a specific configuration of power that needs to be corrected than a dynamic that refers to the aforementioned aporia of the political, which does not exclude – of course – the relevance of thinking of the variations in the contingency, quite the contrary.

It is interesting that Rancière suggests a conceptual variation, a modification in the ways of understanding this dynamic of allocation and appearance that characterizes disagreement.

Politics, from his perspective, is not the sphere of fixation and hierarchical organization, the activity of only delimiting contours and areas inherent to a grouping, but the moment when all that breaks and is called into question. Hence, the term "politics" is reserved for those moments when an instance that questions order emerges, that is, when something bursts into and shows certain players' capacity of speech, the ability to decisively intervene in the Symbolic, in previously prohibited spaces. Thus, Rancière defines politics as the moment when the part of those that have no part realizes that this sum of the social does not add up and that there is no ultimate sense that justifies their confinement to a degraded position. In other words, politics is left on the side of the Real, of the expression of the disagreement that constitutes the Symbolic:

> Politics exists when the natural order of domination is interrupted by the institution of a part of those that have no part. This institution is the whole of politics as a specific form of connection. It defines the common of the community as a political community, in other words, as divided, as based on a wrong that escapes the arithmetic of exchange and reparation. Beyond this set-up there is no politics. There is only the order of domination or the disorder of revolt.
>
> (1999, p. 12)

Rancière does not carry his notion of politics outside of the Symbolic dimension. It is clear that the inherently political moment, which resembles the revolt, continues to be Symbolic. This is not only because it is an expression of the disagreement, a fault in one way of allocating roles and expectations, but also because the interruption always seeks to inscribe itself in that space, to speak, to say other words, to be heard. So here there is a correct delimitation of the matter, but as we will observe later, it is that destiny of the revolt that explains its non-institutional, or non-organizational, perspective of politics. In Rancière's view, politics does not appear as a Real that suspends order; it is that moment when, seen from the Symbolic, something emerges that discusses the exclusions and shows the abjection, that is, the lack of the lack. Politics is the Real that eats away the order and manifests itself by producing a crisis of the order.

This explains why, in Rancière's view, politics is always politics of equality and emancipation, and not the direction of a space of representation, as Laclau would say. The point, then, that interests Rancière is that instant when definitions, hierarchies, and locations appear to be imposed. That is why it is the displaced who must rise with the aim of manifesting their appreciation of what is white and what is black; that is to say, it is they who must use their capacity to speak since they have been the damaged, the invisibilized. This event is precisely the peak moment of political nature for Rancière. It is a question of what is encapsulated in the oblique, in which he argues that the One of community is divided and does not exist as such. The part of those that have no part expresses that Real of the non-sexual relation that Lacan discussed, that is, the empty place.

Politics is equal to equality precisely because the emergence of those that have no part shows a difference of allocation caused by the "significant masters". Hence, Rancière's work attempts not only to highlight the evident matter of the conflictive nature of the social but also to understand what is emphasized in every constitution of community. Rancière's discourse allows us to observe the knotting that occurs in every community between the emergence of the Real, the presupposed ethical horizon – which is also in the order of the Imaginary – and a specific allocation of roles. In this sense, politics is related to aesthetics and aesthetics to politics. In fact, the whole problem I have commented on regarding disagreement refers to the notion of "distribution of the sensible", which is inserted in such a domain:

> I call the distribution of the sensible the system of self-evident facts of sense perception that simultaneously discloses the existence of something in common and the delimitations that define the respective parts and positions within it. A distribution of the sensible therefore establishes at one and the same time something common that is shared and exclusive parts. This apportionment of parts and positions is based on a distribution of spaces, times, and forms of activity that determines the very manner in which something in common lends itself to participation and in what way various individuals have a part in this distribution.
>
> (2011, p. 12)

Thus, there are policies of aesthetics that question the given world, the world that is presented to us as given, and which additionally help to show, through aesthetics, the artistic interventions in this world, but all this proposes a certain retreat of politics, as if, similarly to what happens with the police, politics for Rancière was only of the register of intervention in art. In both fields – which are one and the same for Rancière – the interruption sets the symbolic inscription in motion. But there is a difference here, for politics must live with it, to such an extent that it is the other thing and not the negation of the police. It would seem then that, faced with this fatal destiny, Rancière sees in aesthetics a less fatalist or a less condemned form of emancipation, but one that is also softer, of a lesser impact. Thus, in the last section of this chapter, I would like to solely focus on how he presents this moment of inscription, which will cease to be egalitarian and emancipatory, that is, political. The abject shall cease to be so to be a new part that is not a part, which again reveals the symbolic impossibility with its effects of meaning.[1]

On this point, it is useful to recall Rancière's famous distinction between "politics" and "police", which expresses a true tension, a non-relation, rather than an opposing relation. I will transcribe both definitions exactly as they appear in the 1995 text:

a)

> Politics is generally seen as the set of procedures whereby the aggregation and consent of collectivities is achieved, the organization of powers, the distribution of places and roles, and the systems for legitimizing this distribution. I propose to give this system of distribution and legitimization another name. I propose to call it the *police*.
>
> (1999, p. 28)

b)

> I now propose to reserve the term politics for an extremely determined activity antagonistic to policing: whatever breaks with the tangible configuration whereby parties and parts or lack of them are defined by a presupposition that, by definition, has no place in that configuration-that of the part of those that have no part. This break is manifest in a series of actions that reconfigure the space where parties, parts, or lack of parts have been defined. Political activity is whatever shifts a body from the place assigned to it or changes a place's destination. It makes visible what had no business being seen, and makes heard a discourse where once there was only place for noise; it makes understood as discourse what was once only heard as noise.
>
> (1999, p. 29)

As an example of politics, Rancière quotes the famous case of the Aventine Secession (287 BC). This event, at the dawn of the Roman republic, allowed the plebeians to obtain a representation in the nascent legal-political order of the city. In Rancière's perspective, it was a clear case of irruption that later, after "the great" sent a negotiator, became part of the community horizon; in Rancière's words, it went from being the order of the political to being the order of the police.

With their departure to the edges of the city, with the abandonment by the dominated of the places allocated by the dominating, the Roman tribes questioned order:

> The story presents us with these two scenes and shows us the two observers and emissaries moving about between them – in only one direction, of

> course. These are atypical patricians who have come to see and hear what is going on in this staging of a nonexistent right. And they observe this incredible phenomenon: the plebeians have actually violated the order of the city. They have given themselves names. They have carried out a series of speech acts linking the life of their bodies to words and word use. In short, in Ballanche's terms, from being "mortals" they have become "men" that is, beings engaging in a collective destiny through words. They have become beings who may very well make promises and draw up contracts.
> (1999, p. 25)[2]

Those who had no part did not barricade themselves as slaves; instead, they did something unthinkable:

> They establish another order, another partition of the perceptible, by constituting themselves not as warriors equal to other warriors but as speaking beings sharing the same properties as those who deny them these. They thereby execute a series of speech acts that mimic those of the patricians: they pronounce imprecations and apotheoses; they delegate one of their number to go and consult their oracles; they give themselves representatives by rebaptizing them. In a word, they conduct themselves like beings with names. Through transgression, they find that they too, just like speaking beings, are endowed with speech that does not simply express want, suffering, or rage, but intelligence. They write, Ballanche tells us, "a name in the sky": a place in the symbolic order of the community of speaking beings, in a community that does not yet have any effective power in the city of Rome.
> (1999, p. 24)[3]

The plebeians established a new horizon in not seeking to insert themselves in that which had been laid out by the patricians. In that context, they did not simply demand that they be considered like them; they sought to manage that space of the sensible that appeared as common but not homogeneous. This shows that the social players share, indefectibly, certain signifiers that inform them, as ultimately "patricians" and "plebeians" were Roman. The interesting point here is the articulation between the instances of politicization and de-politicization that take shape within the context of a society. Egalitarian actions in the use of words impact the order of the sensible: Rome went from an aristocratic republic to a popular republic. Precisely in that moment of inclusion, in that moment enabled by negotiation, there emerged a point of agreement between the excluded and the dominant sectors; there appeared, in Rancière's words, the police logic activating new forms of exclusion. Therefore, the gestation of that process that continuously allocates social roles and places began.

Between politics and police, there is no negation; they are articulated forms of the development of the social. Hence, it is important to note that not every irruption undermines order or is re-inscribed. However, when this does happen, the "police" seeks to take a stance by managing the scopes of such a phenomenon. Its task is to stabilize community life. Although this appears as an analytically negative moment in that it contradicts emancipation, it should not go unnoticed that, in Rancière's own terms, it is something inevitable. Hence, he is far from considering that equality is a difficult path of promotions; there is no possible *Aufhebung*. Politics breaks into that encounter with the police, and it also appears with the police's attempts to encapsulate the Real:

> For a thing to be political, it must give rise to a meeting of police logic and egalitarian logic that is never set up in advance.
>
> So nothing is political in itself. But anything may become political if it gives rise to a meeting of these two logics. The same thing -an election, a strike, a demonstration- can give rise to politics or not give rise to politics. A strike is not political when it calls for reforms rather than a better deal or when it attacks the relationships of authority rather than the inadequacy of wages. It is political when it reconfigures the relationships that determine the workplace in its relation to the community.
>
> (1999, p. 32)

The key factor here is that Rancière dislocates the figure of the One of the community. Hence, his disquisitions can be read explicitly not only against the ideal of the society of consensus that the likes of Jürgen Habermas propose (1984), but also against the ideas of a critic of European Modernity such as Clastres. The disagreement is impossible to eliminate not because of a specific failure of a certain order, the lack of rationality of its players, or political dominance, but because of an ontological gap. For this reason, the meeting between the logic of the police and the logic of politics is never perfect: between "politics" and "police", there is no "sexual relation" either. That One of the community as a whole, that space of the undivided social, is necessarily fractured. It exists as an imaginary, mythical suture; it exists only by knowing that the Real expresses itself and that it fragments, divides, and agitates.

Nonetheless, the works that I have reviewed in this last chapter show that, in political terms, *there is only One*. In the case of Clastres, there only exists that One that still blocks the possibility of a two and that administers the difference by turning certain subjects into truly cursed beings; in the case of Rancière, although the police logic has the emancipatory logic as reverse, it is in the meeting between both that ever-conflictive politics is born, where the division that makes up the One is seen. To put it clearer, there is only One provided that that which is-by-not-being exists as an element that seeks to be represented in the Other; an Other that, in turn, expresses how things should be and designates what its incorrectness is, but which is not, does not exist.

A work like *Disagreement* shows the alterity and the hole of the political; that same hole that was seen with Schmitt from the reversibility of the legal-political categories and the impossibility of the decision, but also from the external threat. Hence, when I state here that there "only is One", it is to indicate that the problem of unity and the common continues to be the crucial problem of the political.

Notes

1 I consider it necessary to continue exploring this point, perhaps in subsequent works, for my notion on abjection does not assert something entirely "new", that is, the expression of something that lacks symbolic inscription and historical sedimentations – all my discussion with Benjamin is based on this point. On the contrary, the abject is a metaphor of the structural lack – something that exceeds the excluded by a specific order and refers to that point where the Symbolic collapses.

2 Similarly to the argument developed in *Disagreement,* Rancière shows an example of "non-place" of the word in *The Names of History: On the Poetics of Knowledge* [1992]. There he comments on the revolt of the legions of Pannonia as from the analysis of Tacitus and the reading of the philologist Erich Auerbach. He is particularly interested in highlighting that it is Percennius – a legionnaire skilled in the use of words – who started to spread intrigue among his comrades.

3 The contiguity with the notion of parrhesia analyzed by Foucault (2014) is notable.

Afterword

At this point, I would like to recap.

Concerned with the autonomy of the political, in my previous investigations, I dealt with a moment of contemporary thinking when this concern took on the utmost importance. I concentrated, more specifically, on the European interwar period, observing certain concessions based on positivist and economicist premises. I returned to conceptual underpinnings on the liberal forms of government, seeking to highlight the role that violence played in social life. So it was that I proposed to navigate through the work of Carl Schmitt and Antonio Gramsci – that is, a Catholic jurist who joined the Nazi party and a leader of the Italian Communist Party who was incarcerated by Benito Mussolini – looking at questions that emphasized the relevance of asking about the political, about that field that is apparently autonomous and, at the same time, tensioned and conditioned by others.[1]

I established, then, a "counterpoint" between Schmitt and Gramsci. I selected certain topics that, one way or another, enabled me to reconstruct their views, which were so dissimilar, so diverse, yet so attentive to certain marks of the era. I tried, in turn, to develop an interpretation that would enable me to review certain dilemmas inherent to a different context than that of these authors, permeated by the imperatives of a globalized world and by the consumer culture that prides itself on forgetting the breaks in its history. One of the evident limits of this work lay in that it did not allow me to note the ultimate background that marked the differences imposed by every hermeneutic task. Subsequently, I considered widening the scope of my research and going beyond the endeavor of understanding the actions of certain de-politicizing discourses that had operated in the first half of the twentieth century. I gradually began analyzing other thematizations that warned about the grounds of the social field, the dangers of essentialisms, and identity closures. For this reason, between that first book, which was limited to the problem of the autonomy of the political, and this one, which is about to conclude, about the ontology of the political, there is not only a pronounced difference but also a continuity: Today, as yesterday, it is a question of the problem of the political, the problem of unity.

DOI: 10.4324/9781003457022-14

Coming across Lacan's work was crucial to advance on this path. It even meant an additional challenge: to articulate psychoanalysis with political theory. The first thing I found here was that Lacan could not be translated just like that, without certain reminders about what translation entails. Lacan, who developed his teaching for clinical practice, had to be mobilized in my own reflection. The three registers of experience enabled me to review certain contemporary disquisitions that, one way or another, metaphorize the lack, watch over that hole of reality – which is, certainly, a sign of our post-foundational time – and to proceed with my concerns about the nature of the political field.

In doing so, it became evident that showing the void of the political leaves any reflection in an aporia that compels us to inquire whether it is feasible for the theory to challenge the contradictions of its own epochal context if there is not a marked difference between theory and practice, in spite of what Kant said.

I believe that the exercise of thinking political with psychoanalysis can be broadened by understanding not only the study of other discourses whose communicational impact and inscription in common sense are notable but also by rethinking some of the most evident and urgent theoretical problems of the last decades of the Western world. In this regard, there is still ample scope with regard to the study of political identifications, subjectivation processes, the bond between the individual and the collective, the singular and the common, but also in relation to ethics, an ethics that not only faces order or thinks how to resist it, its disparagements, and its exclusion processes. An ethics that assumes the clashing nature of the conflict without ultimate resolution beyond its empiric crystallizations and its circumstantial resolutions. To use one last analogy, and also thinking about the future of this research, I would argue that it is a question of thinking of a political ethics that revolves around Creon and not only around Antigone, or, to be fairer, one that reflects on what of Antigone exists in Creon and what of Creon exists in Antigone. Thus, perhaps, the question of order may take on other nuances and make room for new questions.

As we know, in Sophocles' *Oedipus Rex*, the character of Creon is the one who seconds Layo in his reign at Thebes. After the latter's death, at the hands of Oedipus, Creon must take charge of the *polis* but is unable to defeat the Sphinx that torments it. It is Oedipus who achieves this by solving the Sphinx's riddles. Time passes, and after the outbreak of a plague that decimates the inhabitants again, Oedipus, now king, discovers his truth and goes into exile. His destiny is that of Thebes; his destiny is to pay for the guilt of committing parricide unwittingly, not consciously. Thus, he saves the city, once again, at the expense of his personal suffering. Afterwards, Creon must take charge of the city for the second time, at least until the sons of the cursed hero – Eteocles and Polynices – are able to rule. When they are, the brothers take turns in the judiciary of the polis until they quarrel and go to war against each other. They kill each other on the battlefield. Creon then retakes the office of supreme authority, once again dealing with the terrible contingence.

It has become clear that there is little Creon can do to bear the blows of fortune. This is perhaps his greatest tragedy, one that explains less about why he is prevented from being a hero and much more why it is an example of the tragedy that operates at the very heart of the political. The times never smile on Creon.

We may recall that after the death of her brothers, Antigone actively intervenes against the laws to ensure the proper burial of Polynices, who had searched for allies in another polis to attack his, Thebes, thus seeking to defeat Eteocles and his army. Polynices is, in the eyes of the city, a traitor; he cannot be buried with the corresponding funeral, with any kind of honors or recognition, whether public or private. Antigone breaches these laws, buries Polynices, and suffers the worst consequences. Haemon, Antigone's fiancé, son of Creon, blames his father and plots to murder him for his beloved's death. However, he fails in that endeavor and decides to take his own life. His mother, Eurydice, in seeing the corpse of her firstborn son, decides to take the same path to the underworld. Creon shall be henceforth condemned to living without his wife and son, again taking charge of the acephalous *polis*, decimated by the deaths and murders of the ruling house. His responsibility obstructs the possibility of choosing to take his own life or of accompanying his relatives and loved ones in the kingdom of Hades. In Creon, hence, there is an ethics that assumes the lack seeking to sustain the world, a world without ultimate foundation.

Is the life of this Greek character not the most suitable metaphor of politics and of a world that no longer has room for heroes, except for those responsible men and women who must balance the tribulations of the social despite themselves and their own interests, always tending to their convictions, to what is most intimate to them?

Perhaps these questions deserve other pages to continue thinking about politics from a Lacanian perspective. However, they function as an index of what I have sought to highlight from the beginning of this book: The question about the impossible of the order entails an evocation of its importance to making life in society viable and harboring its particularities. The demands, resistances, and criticisms can only be made positive as long as they are part of it, as long as they allow for the realization and updating of a communitarian *ethos*. The content can naturally never be prefixed, not even in theory. It will depend on politics and its power relations and the ways of subjectivizing action.

For this reason, I believe it is in Creon that the relevance of the uniqueness of a character like Antigone takes on importance, and it is in Antigone that the need for an order that contemplates uniqueness and its aspects becomes utterly relevant. In that contamination, there is a gesture that not only links politics with the individual but also shows all its excess in the collective. Politics is the expression of an infinite doing, of a fabric that is made while it is threaded.

Note

1 *Lo político y la derrota. Un contrapunto entre Antonio Gramsci y Carl Schmitt* (2020). Madrid: Guillermo Escolar.

Bibliography

Agamben, G. (1998). *Homo Sacer: Sovereign power and bare life*. Stanford University Press.

Agamben, G. (1999a). *Potentialities: Collected essays in philosophy*. Stanford University Press.

Agamben, G. (1999b). *Remnants of Auschwitz: The witness and the archive. Homo Sacer III*. Zone Books.

Agamben, G. (2005). *State of exception. Homo Sacer II, 1*. The University of Chicago Press.

Agamben, G. (2011). *The kingdom and the glory: For a theological genealogy of economy and government*. Stanford University Press.

Agamben, G. (2015). *Stasis: Civil war as a political paradigm*. Stanford University Press.

Agamben, G. (2021). *Where are we now? The epidemic as politics*. Rowman & Littlefield.

Ahmed, S. (2000). *Strange encounters. Embodied others in post-coloniality*. Routledge.

Ahmed, S. (2004). *The cultural politics of emotion*. Routledge.

Alemán, J. (2014). *Lacan and capitalist discourse neoliberalism and ideology*. Routledge.

Arendt, H. (1972). *Crises of the republic: Lying in politics; civil disobedience; on violence; thoughts on politics and revolution*. Harcourt Brace Jovanovich.

Arendt, H. (1976). *The origins of totalitarianism*. Harcourt Brace Jovanovich.

Arendt, H. (1998). *The human condition*. The University of Chicago Press.

Aristotle. (1995). *The politics of Aristotle*. Oxford University Press.

Aron, R. (1983). *Clausewitz: Philosopher of war*. Routledge.

Badiou, A. (2005). *Being and event*. Continuum.

Badiou, A. (2018). *Lacan: Anti-philosophy 3*. Columbia University Press.

Bataille, G. (1986). *Visions of excess: Selected writings, 1927–1939*. University of Minnesota Press.

Bataille, G. (1993). Abjection and miserable forms. In *More and less*. The MIT Press.

Bendersky, J. (1983). *Carl Schmitt theorist for the Reich*. Princeton University Press.

Benjamin, W. (1979). On language as such and on the language of man. In *One-way street and other writings*. New Left Books.

Benjamin, W. (1986). Fate and character. In *Reflections: Essays, aphorisms, autobiographical writings.* Schocken Books.

Benjamin, W. (2004). *"Toward the Critique of Violence", in Selected Writings. Volume I 1913–1926.* The Belknap Press of Harvard University Press.

Benjamin, W. (2005). *"Capitalism as Religion", in The Frankfurt School's Critique of Religion.* Routledge.

Benjamin, W. (2009). *The Origin of German Tragic Drama.* Verso.

Benjamin, W. (2012). *"Thesis on the Philosophy of History", in Illuminations.* Schocken Books.

Bielefeldt, H. (1998). Carl Schmitt's critique of liberalism: Systematic reconstruction and countercriticism. In D. Dyzenhaus (Ed.), *Law as politics.* University Press.

Blumenberg, H. (1997). Prospect for a theory of nonconceptuality. In *Shipwreck with spectator: Paradigm of a metaphor for existence.* The MIT Press.

Braunstein, N. (2021). *Jouissance. A Lacanian concept.* Suny Press.

Brennan, T. (1993). *History after Lacan.* Routledge.

Brutus, S. J. (1994). *Vindiciae contra Tyrannos.* Cambridge University Press.

Butler, J. (1993). *Bodies that matter: On the discursive limits of "sex".* Routledge.

Butler, J. (1999). *Gender trouble: Feminism and the subversion of identity.* Routledge.

Butler, J. (2000). *Antigone's claim. Kinship between life & death.* Columbia University Press.

Butler, J. (2009). *Frames of war: When is life grievable.* Verso.

Butler, J. (2020). *The force of nonviolence.* Penguin Random House.

Butler, J., Laclau, E., & Žižek, S. (2000). *Contingency, hegemony, universality: Contemporary dialogues on the left.* Verso.

Canguilhem, G. (1978). *On the normal and the pathological.* D. Reidel Publishing Company.

Castoriadis, C. (1987). *The imaginary institution of society.* The MIT Press.

Chow, R. (2006). Sacrifice, mimesis, and the theorizing of victimhood (A speculative essay). *Representations, 94*(1), 131–149.

Clastres, P. (1989). *Society against the state: Essays in political anthropology.* Zone Books.

Clastres, P. (1994). *Archeology of violence.* Semiotext(e).

Clausewitz von, C. (1992). Letter to Fichte. In *Historical and political writings.* Princeton University Press.

Clausewitz von, C. (2007). *On war.* Oxford University Press.

Comay, R. (2020). *Deadlines (literally).* Kingston University.

Copjec, J. (1994). *Supposing the subject,* Verso.

De La Boétie, É. (2015). *The politics of obedience: The discourse of voluntary.* The Mises Institute.

De Maistre, J. (1993). Elucidation on sacrifices. In *St Petersburg dialogue or conversations on the temporal government of providence.* McGill-Queen's University Press.

Deleuze, G., & Guattari, F. (1983). *Anti-Oedipus: Capitalism and schizophrenia.* University of Minnesota Press.

Derrida, J. (1981). Plato's pharmacy. In *Dissemination.* The University of Chicago Press.

Derrida, J. (1992). Force of law: The "mystical foundation of authority". In *Deconstruction and the possibility of justice*. Routledge.
Derrida, J. (1996). *The gift of death*. The University of Chicago Press.
Dolar, M. (1991). "I shall be with you on your wedding-night": Lacan and the uncanny. *October, 58*, 5–23.
Eidelsztein, A. (2009). *The graph of desire: Using the work of Jacques Lacan*. Routledge.
Eribon, D. (2019). *Écrits sur la psychanalyse*. Fayard.
Fisher, M. (2017). *The weird and the eerie*. Repeater Books.
Forsthoff, E. (1934). *Der totale Staat*. Hanseatische Verlagsanstalt.
Foucault, M. (1988). *Technologies of the self: A seminar with Michel Foucault*. University of Massachusetts Press.
Foucault, M. (2014). *On the government of the living: Lectures at the Collège de France, 1979–1980*. Palgrave Macmillan.
Freud, S. (1961). Civilization and its discontents. In *The standard edition of the complete psychological works of Sigmund Freud, Volume XXI (1927–1931): The future of an illusion, civilization and its discontents, and other works*. Hogarth Press/Institute of Psycho-Analysis.
Freud, S. (1981). The "Uncanny". In *The standard edition of the complete psychological works of Sigmund Freud, Volume XVII (1917–1919). An infantile neurosis and other works*. Hogarth Press/Institute of Psycho-Analysis.
Freud, S. (2001). *Totem y Taboo*. Routledge.
Girard, R. (1986). *The scapegoat*. Johns Hopkins University Press.
Girard, R. (1989). *Violence and sacred*. The Johns Hopkins University Press.
Girard, R. (2010). *Battling to the end. Conversations with Benoît Chantre*. Michigan State University Press.
Gramsci, A. (2011). *Prison notebooks*. Columbia University Press.
Habermas, J. (1984). *Theory of communicative action, volume one: Reason and the rationalization of society*. Beacon Press.
Hamacher, W. (1991). Afformative, strike. *Cardozo Law Review, 13*(4), 1133–1157.
Hardt, M., & Negri, A. (2004). *Multitude: War and democracy in the age of empire*. Penguin Books.
Hegel, G. (2003). *Elements of the philosophy of right*. Cambridge University Press.
Heidegger, M. (1977). The word of Nietzsche: "God is dead". In *The question concerning technology and other essays*. Harper and Row.
Hirsch, A. K., & McIvor, D. W. (Eds.). (2019). *The democratic arts of mourning. Political theory and loss*. Lexington Books.
Hobbes, T. (1998). *Leviathan*. Oxford University Press.
Hubert, H., & Mauss, M. (1964). *Sacrifice its nature and function*. The University of Chicago Press.
Jameson, F. (1977). Imaginary and symbolic in Lacan: Marxism, psychoanalytic criticism, and the problem of the subject. *Yale French Studies, 55/56*, 338–395.
Jesi, F. (2000). *Spartakus. Simbologia della rivolta*. Bollati Boringhieri.
Jouhandeau, M. (2006). *De l'abjection*. Gallimard.
Jünger, E. (1993). Total mobilization. In *The Heidegger controversy. A critical reader*. The MIT Press.

Jünger, E. (2007). *The worker: Dominion and form*. Northwestern University Press.
Kafka, F. (2008). *Metamorphosis and other stories*. Penguin Classic.
Kalyvas, A. (2000). Hegemonic sovereignty: Carl Schmitt, Antonio Gramsci and the constituent prince. *Journal of Political Ideologies*, *5*(3), 343–376.
Kalyvas, A. (2008). *Democracy and the politics of the extraordinary: Max Weber, Carl Schmitt, Hannah Arendt*. Cambridge University Press.
Kirwan, M. (2009). *Girard and theology*. T&T Clark.
Kojève, A. (1980). *Introduction to the reading of Hegel: Lectures on the phenomenology of spirit*. Cornell University Press.
Kristeva, J. (1980). *Desire in language: A semiotic approach to literature and art*. Columbia University Press.
Kristeva, J. (1982). *Powers of horror. An essay on abjection*. Columbia University Press.
Kristeva, J. (1984). *Revolution in poetic language*. Columbia University Press.
Kristeva, J. (1991). *Strangers to ourselves*. Columbia University Press.
Kristeva, J. (1998). The subject in process. In *The Tel Quel reader*. Routledge.
Kristeva, J. (2002). *Intimate revolt*. Columbia University Press.
Lacan, J. (1971). *The seminars of Jacques Lacan. Book XVIII: On a discourse that might not be a semblance*. Unpublished.
Lacan, J. (1974–1975). *The seminars of Jacques Lacan. Book XXII: RSI*. Unpublished.
Lacan, J. (1990). *The seminars of Jacques Lacan. Book VII: The Ethics of Psychoanalysis*. W. W. Norton & Company.
Lacan, J. (1998). *The seminars of Jacques Lacan. Book XI: The four fundamental concepts of psychoanalysis*. W. W. Norton.
Lacan, J. (2006a). The function and field of speech and language in psychoanalysis. In *Ecrits: The first complete edition in English*. W. W. Norton.
Lacan, J. (2006b). The instance of the letter in the unconscious, or reason since Freud. In *Ecrits: The first complete edition in English*. W. W. Norton.
Lacan, J. (2006c). The mirror stage as formative of the function as revealed in psychoanalytic experience. In *Ecrits: The first complete edition in English*. W. W. Norton.
Lacan, J. (2006d). The subversion of the subject and the dialectic of desire in the Freudian unconscious. In *Ecrits: The first complete edition in English*. W. W. Norton.
Lacan, J. (2007). *The seminars of Jacques Lacan. Book XVII: The other side of psychoanalysis*. W. W. Norton & Company.
Lacan, J. (2014). *The seminars of Jacques Lacan. Book X: Anxiety*. Polity Press.
Lacan, J. (2018). *The Seminar of Jacques Lacan, Book XIX: . . . or worse*. W. W. Norton & Company.
Lacan, J. (2019). *The seminars of Jacques Lacan. Book VI: Desire and its interpretation*. W. W. Norton & Company.
Laclau, E. (2004). Glimpsing the future. In S. Critchley & O. Marchart (Eds.), *Laclau. A critical reader*. Routledge.
Laclau, E. (2005). *On populist reason*. Verso.
Laclau, E. (2007). Bare life or social indeterminacy? In M. Calarco & S. DeCaroli (Eds.), *Giorgio Agamben: Sovereignty and life*. Stanford University Press.

Laleff Ilieff, R. (2020). *Lo político y la derrota. Un contrapunto entre Antonio Gramsci y Carl Schmitt.* Guillermo Escolar.

Laleff Ilieff, R. (2021). *Poderes de la abyección. Política y ontología lacaniana I.* Miño y Dávila.

Lefort, C. (1988). *Democracy and political theory.* University of Minnesota Press.

Lefort, C. (2019). Democracy and representation. In *The constructivist turn in political representation.* Edinburgh University Press.

Levi, P. (2003). *If this is a man.* Abacus Books.

Liddell Hart, B. (2012). *Strategy: The indirect approach.* Pentagon Press.

Losurdo, D. (1991). *La comunità, la morte, l'Occidente. Heidegger e l'ideologia della guerra.* Bollati Boringhieri.

Marchart, O. (2007). *Post-foundational political thought. Political difference in Nancy, Lefort, Badiou and Laclau.* Edinburgh University Press.

Mccormick, J. (1999). *Carl Schmitt's critique of liberalism: Against politics as technology.* Cambridge University Press.

Mcgowan, T. (2013). *Enjoying what we don't have. The political project of psychoanalysis.* University of Nebraska Press.

Mcgowan, T. (2019). *Emancipation after Hegel: Achieving a contradictory revolution.* Columbia University Press.

Mcivor, D. (2016). *Mourning in America. Race and the politics of loss.* Cornell University Press.

Mehring, R. (2014). *Carl Schmitt: A biography.* Polity Press.

Miller, J.-A. (1988). Extimité. *Prose Studies, 11*(3), 121–131.

Milner, J.-C. (2007). *Les Noms indistincts.* Verdier.

Milner, J.-C. (2021). *A search for clarity: Science and philosophy in Lacan's Oeuvre.* Northwestern University Press.

Moi, T. (1991). *The Kristeva reader.* Basil Blackwell.

Moreiras, A. (2010). Spanish Guerrillas against Napoleon: Political intensity and the world spirit. *Journal of Spanish Cultural Studies, 11*, 3–4.

Palti, E. (2017). *An archeology of the political: Regimes of power from the seventeenth century to the present.* Columbia University Press.

Paret, P. (1985). *Clausewitz and the state: The man, his theories, and his times.* Princeton University Press.

Paret, P. (2015). Machiavelli, Fichte, and Clausewitz in the Labyrinth of German idealism. *Ethics & Politics, XVII*(3), 78–95.

Parker, I., & Pavón-Cuéllar, D. (2021). *Psychoanalysis and revolution: Critical psychology for liberation movements.* 1968 Press.

Plato. (2003). *The republic.* Cambridge University Press.

Plato. (2008). *Timaeus and Critias.* Penguin Classics.

Preterossi, G. (2022). *Political theology and law.* Routledge.

Rancière, J. (1991). *The ignorant schoolmaster: Five lessons in intellectual emancipation.* Stanford University Press.

Rancière, J. (1994). *The names of history: On the poetics of knowledge.* University of Minnesota Press.

Rancière, J. (1999). *Disagreement: Politics and philosophy.* University of Minnesota Press.

Rancière, J. (2011). *The politics of aesthetics: The distribution of the sensible.* Continuum.

Roudinesco, E. (1997). *Jacques Lacan*. Columbia University Press.
Sabsay, L. (2016). *The political imaginary of sexual freedom*. Palgrave.
Santner, E. (2005). Miracles happen: Benjamin, Rosenzweig, Freud, and the matter of the neighbor. In K. Reinhard, E. L. Santner, & S. Zizek (Eds.), *The neighbor: Three inquiries into political theology*. The University of Chicago Press.
Schmitt, C. (1967). Clausewitz als politischer Denker. Bemerkungen und Hinweise. *Der Staat*, *6*(4), 479–502.
Schmitt, C. (1986). *Political romanticism*. MIT Press.
Schmitt, C. (1988). *Political theology: Four chapters on the concept of sovereignty*. The MIT Press.
Schmitt, C. (1994). Totaler Feind, totaler Krieg, totaler Staat. In *Positionen und Begriffe im Kampf mit Weimar – Genf – Versailles. 1923–1939*. Duncker & Humblot.
Schmitt, C. (2004). *Theory of the partisan: Intermediate commentary on the concept of the political*. Telos Press Publishing.
Schmitt, C. (2006). *Nomos of the earth in the international law of the Jus Publicum Europaeum*. Telos Press.
Schmitt, C. (2007). *The concept of the political*. The University of Chicago Press.
Schmitt, C. (2008). *Constitutional theory*. Duke University Press.
Schmitt, C. (2015). *Land and sea: A world-historical meditation*. Telos Press Publishing.
Schmitt, C. (2016). *Der Hüter der Verfassung*. Duncker & Humblot.
Schmitt, C. (2017). *Ex Captivitate Salus: Experiences 1945–47*. Polity Press.
Schmitt, C. (2018). *The Tyranny of values and other*. Telos Press.
Sophocles. (2006). *Oedipus rex*. Cambridge University Press.
Sorel, G. (1999). *Reflections on violence*. Cambridge University Press.
Stavrakakis, Y. (2000). *Lacan and the political*. Routledge.
Stavrakakis, Y. (2007). *The Lacanian left psychoanalysis, theory, politics*. Edinburgh University Press/SUNY Press.
Stavrakakis, Y. (Ed.). (2020). *Routledge handbook of psychoanalytic political theory*. Routledge.
Strauss, L. (1995). Notes on Carl Schmitt *The concept of the political*. In H. Meier (Ed.), *Carl Schmitt and Leo Strauss: The hidden dialogue*. The University of Chicago Press.
Tönnies, F. (2001). *Community and civil society*. Cambridge University Press.
Tse-Tung, M. (2007). On contradiction. In *On practice and contradiction*. Verso.
Von Ludendorff, E. (1936). *The nation at war*. Hutchinson.
Weber, M. (2004). *The vocation lectures*. Hackett Publishing Company.
Williams, J. (2000). *The Girard reader*. Crossroad Herder.
Zafiropoulos, M. (2001). *Lacan et les sciences sociales-le déclin du pere (1938–1953)*. PUF.
Žižek, S. (2000). *The ticklish subject: The absent centre of political ontology*. Verso.
Žižek, S. (2002). *Welcome to the desert of the real!* Verso.
Žižek, S. (2008). *Violence: Six sideways reflections*. PICADOR.
Žižek, S. (2013). *Less than nothing: Hegel and the shadow of dialectical materialism*. Verso.
Zupančič, A. (2008). *Why psychoanalysis? Three interventions*. NSU Press.

Index

Note: Page numbers in *italic* indicate a figure on the corresponding page.

For Product Safety Concerns and Information please contact our EU representative GPSR@taylorandfrancis.com
Taylor & Francis Verlag GmbH, Kaufingerstraße 24, 80331 München, Germany

www.ingramcontent.com/pod-product-compliance
Lightning Source LLC
LaVergne TN
LVHW010927110826
845149LV00013B/2507
9781032599687